The Use of Group Services in Permanency Planning for Children

The *Social Work with Groups* series

Series Editors: Catherine P. Papell and Beulah Rothman

- *Co-Leadership in Social Work with Groups,* Beulah Rothman and Catherine P. Papell
- *Social Groupwork & Alcoholism,* Marjorie Altman and Ruth Crocker, Guest Editors
- *Group Work with the Frail Elderly,* Shura Saul, Guest Editor
- *The Use of Group Services in Permanency Planning for Children,* Sylvia Morris, Guest Editor
- *Activities and Action in Groupwork,* Ruth Middleman, Guest Editor
- *Gender in Groupwork,* Charles Garvin and Beth Reed, Guest Editors
- *Ethnicity in Groupwork Practice,* Larry Davis, Guest Editor
- *Time as a Factor in Groupwork,* Albert Alissi and Max Casper, Guest Editors
- *Groupwork with Children & Adolescents,* Ralph Kolodny and James Garland, Guest Editors
- William Schwartz memorial issue (title to be announced), Alex Gitterman and Lawrence Shulman, Guest Editors

The Use of Group Services in Permanency Planning for Children

Sylvia Morris
Guest Editor

The Haworth Press
New York

The Use of Group Services in Permanency Planning for Children has also been published as *Social Work with Groups*, Volume 5, Number 4, Winter 1982.

The Haworth Press, Inc., 28 East 22 Street, New York, NY 10010

Library of Congress Cataloging in Publication Data
Main entry under title:

The Use of group services in permanency planning for children.

(Social Work with groups ; v. 5. no. 4)
Includes bibliographies.
1. Social work with children—United States—Addresses, essays, lectures. 2. Social group work—Addresses, essays, lectures. 3. Foster home care—United States—Addresses, essays, lectures. I. Morris, Sylvia. II. Series: Social work with groups (Haworth Press) ; v. 5, no. 4.
HV45.S63 vol. 5, no. 4 [HV741] 361.4s [362.7] 82-23389
ISBN 0-86656-199-4

The Use of Group Services in Permanency Planning for Children

Social Work with Groups
Volume 5, Number 4

CONTENTS

BOOK REVIEWS

AUDIO-VISUAL REVIEW

HELEN NORTHERN, PhD, *School of Social Work, University of Southern California, Los Angeles*
RUBY B. PERNELL, DSW, *School of Applied Social Sciences, Case Western Reserve University, Cleveland*
HELEN PHILLIPS, DSW, *School of Social Work, University of Pennsylvania, Philadelphia*
HERMAN RESNICK, PhD, *School of Social Work, University of Washington, Seattle*
SHELDON ROSE, PhD, *School of Social Work, University of Wisconsin, Madison*
JANICE H. SCHOPLER, MSW, *Assistant Professor, School of Social Work, University of North Carolina, Chapel Hill*
MARY LOUISE SOMERS, DSW, *School of Social Service Administration, University of Chicago*
EMANUEL TROPP, MSSW, *School of Social Work, Virginia Commonwealth University, Richmond*
ROBERT VINTER, PhD, *School of Social Work, University of Michigan, Ann Arbor*
CELIA B. WEISMAN, DSW, *Wurzweiler School of Social Work, Yeshiva University, New York*
GERTRUDE WILSON, MA, *University of California, Berkeley*

The Use of Group Services in Permanency Planning for Children

EDITORIAL

Permanency planning offers the opportunity to review and re-establish the presence of group work in child welfare services. The history of group work practice in child welfare dates back to the post-World War II period when there was an upsurge of professionally led group services offered in the voluntary sector of all social welfare programs.

In child welfare, demonstration projects serving children in care began to utilize the growing professional skill of social group workers. Group services designed to meet the developmental needs of children in foster care were introduced. Group workers were also called upon to organize programs which would enable foster parents to extend and improve their nurturing abilities and to create mutual aid for the critical and demanding care of children placed in their homes. Group workers were asked to train child care workers and other child welfare staff to sensitize them to group dynamics and natural group interactions as means for growth and coping. In the emerging establishment of small group homes in the community, group work practitioners often introduced the disciplined use of democratic participation in group governance.

Group work efforts in all of these situations concentrated on supporting the children in placement, attending to their emotional health and social growth needs on the one hand, and on the other hand, humanizing the foster care system. Less consideration was given to group services that would ultimately move children out of foster care and into their homes of origin or permanent placement, although there were some experimental programs, such as one which an editor of this journal helped to develop for natural parents and children in placement.[1] Other group programs, foreshadowing the present focus on permanency, were related to adoption, and services for the care of unmarried teenage mothers. However, the foster care system, including the full range of residential and community patterns, seemed to be the permanent structure providing interim to long-term maintenance and protection for dependent children.[2] Permanency planning in the '80s has redefined the situation changing the philosophical and legal premises for child welfare.

Group work can respond accordingly. These editors see the issue of permanency as a stimulus to focusing attention on child welfare as a major domain for effective social group work service. In its early origins, group work began by offering services to children. It has never lost its commitment. Today's issues require that group services be offered to children in care and to the participants in the caring system whether these be natural parents, adoptive parents, and/or foster parents in order that ultimately all may be enabled to realize a more stable and enduring family life.

Sylvia Morris, our Guest Editor, has been in the forefront of manpower training for child welfare, in public and private agencies. The journal is honored to have her leadership in bringing together these contributors.

CP
BR

REFERENCES

1. Gladys Simmons, Joanne Gumpert, and Beulah Rothmann. "Natural Parents as Partners in Child Placement." *Social Casework, 54* 1973, 224, 232.
2. David Fanschel.

GUEST EDITOR

SYLVIA K. MORRIS, MSW, is a Child Welfare Consultant. She was formerly Deputy Director of Training, New York City Human Resources Administration and Assistant Executive Director, Louise Wise Services, a New York City child welfare agency.

GUEST EDITORIAL

Over the last decade, issues of permanency planning for children have been given nationwide attention by the professional and civic communities. The interfacing of the social service and court systems, coupled with the overriding concern of violence and crime in the urban areas, has catapulted this movement into the public limelight. This has been reinforced and stimulated by the general interest in deinstitutionalization and the specific concern for mounting costs of the foster care system. In a New York *Times* series entitled "Rights of Children, A Decade of Change," Collins reported:

> The Federal Government spends nearly $1 billion for children in out-of-home care as part of the Child Welfare Services Program, The Foster Care Program, Title XX of the Social Security Act and other programs. Some 20 percent of the 500,000 in foster care are in institutions and group homes, while 100,000 are in the mental health, special education and other institutions according to estimates of the Census Bureau and other agencies.[1]

The mean length of stay for children placed out-of-home before the age of 2 is seven years.

While emphasis in federal spending is shifting to protective and preventive services, many who work for child welfare reform fear the consequences of the federal budget cutbacks. It is now highly politicized. Lack of crucial supports will have a demonstratable effect on vulnerable families. Not only may more new children be at risk of coming into the child welfare system, but those families prepared to reunite with children in placement will be under far greater strain because of cuts in food stamps, medical payments, special education programs, etc. Efforts at permanency have always been an underlying concern of the social work profession. Realization that a child in the foster care systems is basically a child of the "system" has propelled us to take even more aggressive steps towards reunification and adoption. With the recessive state of the economy, it will require using all available resources and service modalities to accomplish this goal.

Social case work, historically, has been the core service provided in adoption and foster care. Staff of child welfare agencies have been recruited with this training in mind. This needs to be aggressively reassessed.

This issue, "The Use of Group Services in Permanency Planning," only begins to address the need for broader perspectives in program directions and manpower development. The papers presented in this edition reflect and describe the impact of the relationship of federal to state and local programs. The trend of this relationship will be more in the nature of consultation, establishment of "consortia" resources, e.g., combination of special expertise to span a spectrum of skills in response to shrinking resources. Group work as a modality is paramount whether the groups are under professional or community leadership, whether they are groups providing direct service, networking, advocacy, organizational planning, or manpower development. The authors of these papers essentially describe these different services. Illustrated also are the real difficulties in this current climate in the provision of services and the obstacles inherent in institutional change coupled with reassessment of service delivery. They do not represent success stories but rather a strong commitment to the integrity of permanency planning concepts and the struggles to achieve this through group process.

The thrust towards research and the development of teaching training materials in this practice area may have reached its peak for the present. Nonetheless, the commitment of creating and maintaining stable and caring environments for children requires the incorporation of group work and family practice as an integral part of child welfare services to be delivered by those who have the appropriate training. Differential use of treatment modalities is not a new concept. The application of group work services in child welfare, as described in this journal, suggests the need for stronger investment in manpower development on the part of program planners. Until that time, we may continue to rely only on the caseworker with the child at the center of the problem without the skills needed to work with families and other associated systems. The full realization of permanency planning cannot succeed without the interactional perspective of the small group as an instrument of change.

Sylvia K. Morris, CSW
May 1982

REFERENCE

1. New York *Times*. "Rights of Children, A Decade of Change." First of a series of articles, July 21, 1981, Glen Collins.

Group Work with Natural Parents in Permanency Planning

I. A Conceptual Framework and Literature Review
II. An Example of a Natural Parent Group

Rosemarie Carbino

ABSTRACT. Group work with parents of children in foster care has good potential as a complement to casework services in permanency planning. An underused social work service in child welfare, group work has rarely been provided to natural parents. It can be utilized differentially along the foster care continuum from needs identification through aftercare to provide parents information, support and training specific to foster care. Reports of group work services for abusing parents, parents of children in residential treatment and special programs for natural parents provide relevant information for design of group work with natural parents. An example of a group of parents whose children are in foster home placement is presented. Special considerations for providing group services to natural parents are highlighted. Group work appears to have positive effects on the providing agency as well as on parent group participants. Issues regarding group work in permanency planning include the risk of its misuse through agency-imposed agendas and/or agency-determined timetables for individual and group development. It will be helpful to study what group services with which parents at which points in the foster care continuum assist permanency planning efforts.

Rosemarie Carbino, MSW, is a clinical assistant professor at the School of Social Work, University of Wisconsin–Madison.

I. A CONCEPTUAL FRAMEWORK AND LITERATURE REVIEW

Introduction

Group work with parents of children in foster care has considerable potential to complement casework services in permanency planning efforts. Although it has been overlooked as a service modality in current practice and policy efforts focused on natural parents, it can produce special benefits for both providers and the consumers of agency foster care services.

This two-part article will focus on the uses of group work with parents in permanency planning services. Section I will present a conceptual framework and literature review. These important areas will be reviewed as background: foster care theory and practice; permanency planning concepts, focusing primarily on public welfare systems; the status of natural parents in foster care, highlighting their special needs; and group work as a social work method in child welfare services. The relevance of group work services for natural parents at various points in the foster care continuum will then be discussed. Finally, literature on related parent groups will be reviewed in terms of its implications for group services to natural parents.

Section II will present an example of group work with parents of children in foster placement to illustrate group work service at one point in the continuum. Considerations relevant to group work with parents in agencies involved in permanency planning will be considered and some issues will be raised.

Foster Care Theory and Practice

Foster care can be defined as the planned, time-limited placement of a minor in a licensed foster family, group home or residential facility, when needed care or services cannot be provided in the child's own family setting. The placement is made under the supervision of a licensed child welfare agency and, in public services, is often accompanied by a transfer of legal custody from the parent(s) to a county or state having jurisdiction.

Foster placement is viewed as one of several child welfare service options. It is a partial means of providing treatment and other services for families and children toward specified goals. It is not intended as an end in itself. Ideally, it is used when selected as the service of choice from a range of others only when concrete support (such as health care) and preventive services to family are unable to help the family maintain the child's well-being in the family setting.

Where foster family care is the selected service, the process can be viewed as a continuum from referral through placement and exit from foster home care.

Potential Family and Child Services
in the Foster Care Continuum

Points in the Foster Care Continuum	*Potential Services*
Identification of needs/problems	Preventive and supportive services.
Referral to foster care	Supportive and crisis intervention services. Exploration of foster care and alternative services.
Intake to foster care	Continued preventive and supportive services, as applicable, for parents and other children. Fuller exploration of foster care. Contracting with all involved parties. (Recontracting continues at all points.)
Placement	Placement services, including foster home visitation, contracting and work on separation and loss. Direct services, related to goals of placement, are begun.
Undercare	Goal-related direct services, including planned visitation, continue. Family supportive services continue.
Exit	Placement services, including visiting, contracting and work on separation and loss. Continuing supportive services. Possible termination services for child and natural family.
Aftercare	Supportive and preventive services.

Along the continuum, there are a number of recommended foster care services for children and their families. These represent what services should be available, rather than what may actually be available. At IDENTIFICATION of any service needs which signal some risk of foster care, there is provision of supportive and preventive services. At REFERRAL to foster care, there are crisis intervention services and supportive services. There may also be exploration of foster care and its alternatives. At INTAKE to foster care, there is a more comprehensive exploration of foster care and contracting with all involved parties for service. Recontracting continues throughout the foster care process. At PLACEMENT, a transitional phase, placement services (including foster home visitation and work on separation and loss) and direct services are provided. In the UNDERCARE phase, the period of time the child is in foster family placement, direct services to child and natural family continue. These include planned visitation and emphasize problem-resolution and environmental support. The EXIT phase, another transitional phase, includes placement services and planning for the child's return home, or alternate permanent placement for the child and termination services for child and family. In AFTERCARE, supportive and/or preventive services are appropriate.

The reality of foster care practice, particularly in the public welfare sector, is that few alternatives may be available (Kadushin, 1980; Stein et al., 1978), that placements are often crisis oriented and unplanned (Sauber, 1967), that few services and poor quality services are rendered to natural parents (Kadushin, 1980; Knitzer and Allen, 1978; Stone, 1969), and that placements may continue much longer than intended (Wiltse, 1976). Progress in system change is slow for a variety of reasons related to public funding priorities and resultant service delivery; the scope of the service need; and the often extremely disadvantaged socioeconomic status of families needing child welfare services.

Permanency Planning

Permanency planning represents a response to a major problem in foster care: the large number of children who continue in placement for years without planned outcomes or stable, continuous placements. Definitions of permanency and emphases in permanency planning projects are varied (Maluccio et al., 1980). Permanency planning will be defined here as a commitment through action by foster care system representatives to ensure a child's sense of continuity and the stability of family relationships by prompt decision-making and intervention at three points. These are (1) preventing inappropriate entry into foster care by provision of alternative services; (2) when foster placement must occur, shortening the time spent in care by giving services to parents or families focused on early reunification of the family; and (3) when return home is not feasible within a specified length of time (usually given as 18-24 months), providing either an alternative permanent placement through adoption and legal termination of parental rights (TPR) and responsibilities or provision of planned, long-term foster home placement, or independent living (Pike, 1976; Stein, 1976; Wiltse, 1976). The rationale of permanency planning is that a child's sense of stability and continuity requires a clear plan for permanency and active interventions to achieve the plan.

A variety of efforts at other levels also focus on reducing foster care and may be viewed as part of the permanency planning impetus. However, this discussion will focus solely on direct agency services to natural families.

Major permanency planning projects have reported success in achieving the desired outcome of decreasing the numbers of children in care by intensive work to provide planned permanent living situations (Pike, 1976; Stein et al., 1978). Depending upon the program emphasis and target population, this might mean returning more children home promptly through intensive family services (Jones, 1976; Stein et al., 1978) or freeing more children for adoption (Pike, 1976). In addition, permanency planning projects report other benefits in worker skills and agency services. However, when some differences in control and experimental samples in reported projects are taken into account, permanency planning activities may not demonstrate high effectiveness over regular agency services in achieving permanent placements (Kadushin, 1980; Maluccio et al., 1980). In addition, it is important to consider whether the achievement of the administrative outcome (permanent placement) does indeed result in the service outcome (child's sense of permanence and stability) since it is possible for children to perceive "temporary" placements as permanent (Lahti et al., 1978). Thus, evaluation of the success of permanency planning will need to continue for some time.

Natural Parents of Children in Foster Care

One intended effect of a permanency planning focus upon agency foster care interventions is earlier and increased attention to natural parents of children in placement. Natural parents, particularly parents of young children, are likely to have an extremely disadvantaged status in society. Many have serious economic, health and/or housing problems (Fanshel, 1978; Kadushin, 1980; Sauber, 1967; Sussman, 1970; Torczyner and Paré, 1979); many are single parents, usually women with little education. Oppressed racial and ethnic minorities are overrepresented in this population (Kadushin, 1980). In addition, the parents are likely to have greater emotional disturbance than parents of children not placed in foster care (Kadushin, 1980), to be lacking familial and community supports (Torczyner and Paré, 1979), and to be in crisis at the time of placement (Sauber, 1967). Thus, the parents may be simultaneously in circumstances which make service delivery both difficult (Fanshel, 1978) and critically needed.

The need for planned, intensive and comprehensive services to natural parents has continuously been affirmed (Child Welfare League of America, 1979; Knitzer and Allen, 1978; Shyne and Schroeder, 1978). Over the years, many projects have demonstrated effective preventive or rehabilitative interventions at various points in the continuum of services (Boyd, 1979; Jones, B., 1964; Jones, M., 1976; Kautz, 1969; Maybanks, 1979; Rubenstein, 1967; Shyne et al., 1972; Stein et al., 1978). Despite the acknowledged need for service and the possibilities for service demonstrated by a number of projects, the actual frequency and quality of services to natural parents are poor (Kadushin, 1980; Stone, 1969). This is particularly true in regard to preventive services, to services for parents whose children have been in placement for several years, and to aftercare services (Stone, 1969).

In addition, parents report their experiences with the foster care system as a whole, including agencies, foster families, other service providers and juvenile court and detention systems, as reinforcing their feelings of being "failures" and isolated outsiders in the system (Carbino, 1981). To quote a parent of placed children:

> I realize foster care is necessary sometimes, but it was just an awful feeling, I felt very like a complete failure and terribly, terribly, hurt. That I had people saying to me that you can't do this, you're not good enough. You're not a fit mother.

Further, natural parents are generally uninformed about agency services, foster care and legal processes and what is expected of them (Carbino, 1981).

Recent efforts in permanency planning are attempting to focus considerable attention on early engagement of parents in joint and intensive effort towards mutually agreed-upon outcomes wherever possible (Stein, 1976). As pointed out earlier, these programs report increases in permanency placements for children. Lacking parent evaluation of the programs, it is not possible to discover if these intensive efforts result in more positive experiences with the foster care system for parents.

The factors of foster care service delivery; natural parent circumstances and characteristics and parent experiences in the foster care system have implications for the design of group work service in permanency planning. These will be discussed in a subsequent section.

Group Work as a Social Work Service in Child Welfare

Group work has long been an appropriate, if underused, complement to casework services in child welfare (American Public Welfare Association, 1962; Child Welfare League of America, 1963; Montelius, 1966). Its particular value for permanency planning is its usefulness as a method to address some of the issues common to many parents of children in or entering foster placement. Its uses in child welfare practice will be examined here with particular attention to relevance for work with parents in permanency planning efforts.

Because of the risks of terminological confusion arising from the proliferation of group intervention procedures in recent years (Lang, 1979), it will be helpful to begin with a brief delineation of what is meant here by group work. We view it as a social work method, rooted in the same values and ethical principles of confidentiality, self-determination and voluntary participation as other social work methods. It uses the small group as both the context and the means of service (Vinter, 1967). The small group offers its members support and a safe place to learn and try out new behaviors and ideas (Glasser, 1963). The outcome goals of group work practice are those of improved personal functioning and/or positive changes in the member's social environment (Vinter, 1967). The social worker's role is as facilitator of the group's development and functioning; it is not a role of individual therapist in group context nor of permanent leader (Lang, 1979). While the group services reviewed herein vary in the degree to which they reflect this group work formulation, they are close enough to be included.

We view group work services in public welfare as underused, particularly in child welfare. Casework is and has been the predominant method of service since the origins of public social services in the 1930s. During the 1960s there was an increasing use of group work services in child welfare agencies, particularly with AFDC mothers' groups (American Public Welfare Association, 1962; Child Welfare League of America, 1963; Montelius, 1966; Navarre et al., 1974). However, that growth has not continued; use of group work appears to have declined. There is little reported current use of group work service in child welfare, with the exception of groups for abusive/neglecting parents, usually mothers (Avery and Wayne, 1978; Belucci, 1972; Breton, 1979; Davoren, 1975; Kruger et al., 1979). Some child management training with AFDC parents in a group context has been described (Rose, 1977).

Group work services in foster care have been used fairly often with foster parents in training and education (Weinbach et al., 1977) and occasionally with foster teenagers (Carter, 1968; Lee and Park, 1978; Peterson and Sturgies, 1971) and pre-adolescents (Ludlow and Epstein, 1972; Watson, 1968). However, they have rarely been used in work with parents (Stone, 1969), with the exceptions of some group programs in residential treatment settings (Heiting, 1971; Magnus, 1974; Simmons et al., 1973; Winder et al., 1965) and occasional special projects (Edinger, 1970; Murphy, 1976).

Group work services for parents can be useful all along the foster care continuum, both in providing basic support and learning experiences and providing specific information, support and training in foster care matters. Specific information could be shared on foster care and permanency planning goals, processes and services; court processes; parent rights and roles; and the respective rights and roles of others. Supportive services are particularly needed through important foster care events such as placement, changes of placement, court hearings, return and TPR. Specific skills training could include areas such as contracting, working with the agency and foster family, visiting, and participating in court hearings.

Group services design and emphasis will, of course, differ depending on parent needs along the continuum. At IDENTIFICATION and REFERRAL, group work service may be used as a preventive effort along with any needed concrete assistance such as housing, food and medical care. At INTAKE to foster care, group experience could offer early support from other parents and much-needed information in a way that parents can "hear" and begin to understand it. At PLACEMENT and through the UNDERCARE phase, group work can offer parents support and information, as well as an opportunity to develop their abilities to function more effectively. In addition, groups here may be able to become effective advocates on behalf of their members and other natural parents. As EXIT from foster care occurs, groups can serve important support functions. Since aftercare services and post-TPR services for parents are infrequent, group services at this point in the continuum might be primary service modes. Thus group work in foster care can be utilized at many points and in a variety of ways to assist parents.

Parent Group Services: A Review of Selected Literature

Reports of actual group work services rendered in several settings have relevance for work with parents of foster children. Group work with abusing parents, in residential programs, and in special programs will be reviewed here.

Group work with abusing parents. The reports of group work with abusive parents (Avery and Wayne, 1978; Belluci, 1972; Breton, 1979; Davoren, 1975; Kruger et al., 1979) evidence a number of parallels to the circumstances of parents of foster children, especially of young children. Abusive parent group members were in seriously disadvantaged circumstances economically, socially and personally. They were isolated, lacking familial and community supports. They were in need of multiple simultaneous services for a host of problems, of which child caring was just one. They were in obvious need of nurture and attention for themselves as well as on behalf of their children.

Group purposes included goals of personal support and growth; increased understanding and ability to care for their children. The groups were small, staffed by social workers. Meeting weekly or twice a month, they lasted over relatively long periods of time, perhaps 12-22 months. Although the amount of information on development of the group process varied in the reports, it was clear that groups remained in pregroup and early group formation stages for a long time.

We note that participants were active and vocal from early on in the group meetings, particularly in sharing problems and ventilating feelings. However, workers found it necessary to take early and continuing responsibility for group development and intensive support to members.

Group outcomes were reported as successful. These anecdotal evaluations from workers, members and observers described reduction in parent isolation, increased understanding of service goals for children, improved personal and social functioning, and improved self-esteem (Avery and Wayne, 1978; Belluci, 1972; Breton, 1979; Kruger et al., 1979; McFerran, 1958). It is unclear how much change occurred in parenting. Another outcome reported was the frequent development of mutual support systems among members outside of the group meetings (Breton, 1979; Kruger et al., 1979).

Group work with parents in residential treatment. Reports of group services to parents of children in residential treatment (Simmons et al., 1973; Winder, 1965) echo the experiences of group work with abusive parents. Parents were in similarly deprived, multiproblem, crisis-ridden circumstances, in need of concrete assistance and nurture. Active and continuous work by group services staff was required; group development and individual member growth took a long time. Parents needed time to share feelings and air complaints. Some positive changes in use of help and in parenting and positive changes in agency response to parents were reported to occur.

Group work with natural parents of foster children. Reports of two group programs for parents of children in foster homes (Edinger, 1970; Murphy, 1976) also show a number of parallels. Though these parents were selected as promising candidates for earlier return of children they evidenced deprivation and considerable emotional need. They used group sessions to ask many questions and air complaints about the agency. They appear, however, to have become involved in the group's development somewhat sooner than members of abusive parent groups, once the initial volume of ventilation of feeling had abated. In addition, they were able to bring group concerns to agency attention and act effectively on behalf of other parents. Both groups pointed out that they experienced considerable negative labeling and treatment by personnel of the foster care system.

Implications for Group Work in Permanency Planning with Natural Parents

These reports of group services have obvious relevance for group work with natural parents in permanency planning efforts. For parents in disadvantaged circumstances, group work can be an excellent means of countering the problems of isolation, of lack of familial and community supports, and of lack of information about the foster care system and their legal rights. At the same time, such parents can be expected to need a number of intensive and simultaneous services. Thus, group service cannot be conceived of as the sole service to be rendered.

Groups for natural parents may well need to provide considerable support and nurture, to be realistic about the slower pace at which the groups can be expected to develop, and to be sensitive and practical in setting goals that relate to members' expressed needs. Group workers can expect that many early meetings will be utilized by individual participants for airing feelings and problems before they are prepared to consider a group focus. Groups are likely to be attended primarily by women; while this reflects the reality of societal structure, it may mean overlooking important potential participants in family change.

Staff of public social service agencies cannot be expected to be experienced group workers. They can learn and succeed in group work with supervision and other agency backing. This includes freeing them from some caseload responsibilities to plan, organize and facilitate the group(s); assurance of concrete services such as transportation and child care for members; and support for the group worker's protection of confidentiality for members. It is our opinion that, in order to avoid role conflict, the group worker should not be simultaneously responsible for casework and case recommendations regarding child and family.

Some group work programs have been influential factors in agency decisions to provide new informational resources for natural family members and/or to provide education to staff about natural parents (Murphy, 1976). Agency policy and practice regarding services and visits have also been influenced (Edinger, 1970; Simmons et al., 1973; Winder et al., 1965). This suggests that interchange with natural parents through group work service can positively influence agency perceptions of and responses to them.

II. AN EXAMPLE OF A NATURAL PARENT GROUP

> We belong to a group where for once we can share our feelings. We can let our hair down. We were in it all alone and you're wondering what you're going to do . . . . You can't talk to the neighbors. It's a blessing that I found the group . . . You have to remember how very tired you were

> after all this struggle. There are other people, I'm sure, who are going through it who are, at this point, very, very tired, exhausted . . . . We all know what one another is feeling and we have this bond. (parent group member)

We will present here, as an illustration of group work with natural parents in the UNDERCARE phase of foster care services, a review of parent group meetings which were part of a larger project to develop a parent organization.[1]

Group Meetings in the Context of the Project

The overall purpose of the project was to develop an association for parents of foster children which might provide information and mutual support and serve as an organized voice on behalf of parents, particularly in improving how the foster care system views and treats them. This organizational effort utilized a small team of social work students, field instructors, an agency staff consultant and a number of natural parents during the two-year period. While parents and staff were involved in a variety of organizational activities including individual and subgroup tasks, the focus here will be solely upon the group meetings as an example of group work with natural parents.

In some ways, the group experience clearly differed from group work as a medium of personal change. The most influential difference was that the outcome goal was building an organization rather than effecting personal change. Other differences were a function of this. Membership was open to all parents with children in substitute care. Size was not limited; parents entered and left throughout the project. Parent members and staff were involved in many business-focused and planning tasks in and outside of group meetings. Parents and staff became actively involved with community professionals whom they viewed both as targets of influence and as helpers. Group meetings regularly included speakers as part of the information-gathering effort.

Yet, the group meetings in many ways reflected basic group work practice and normal group developmental processes. To a great extent, this was because group work services of this nature are usually unavailable to parents of foster children. Thus, within a clear and agreed-upon organizational focus, parents emphasized the mutual support and problem-sharing aspects of the group meetings as an early and continuing priority. Staff worked with the group as a whole and with its members to facilitate the group's development through various phases and to assist it to problem-solve, to make decisions, to strengthen leadership and to set and implement goals.

Group Phases

We will use Hartford's (1971) conceptualization of phases in group development as a way of organizing information on the group experience. Group purposes, membership, developmental processes and group worker roles will be considered.

I. Pregroup Phases: Private, public and convening

The first of three Pregroup Phases is the "private" phase, a period of conceptual recognition of need and group work potential. For purposes of this discussion, it is sufficient to say that the program idea developed from the author's experience with foster parent organizations and with natural parents as presenters in foster care educational programs.

The "public" phase included a period of considerable planning, then recruitment efforts. Because the program was not located within an agency, confidentiality prohibited direct access to potential members. Agencies were asked to inform parents about the program; posters, informational letters and newspaper ads were also used. There was support from agencies and workers as well as agency delays and worker resistance to referral. Meetings were designed to last 2 hours and were held every other week on a weekday evening at a local church; transportation and child care were made available. Speakers on subjects of concern to parents were planned as part of most meetings, along with opportunities for participants to interrelate and share.

In the "convening" phase, potential members meet. There is an aggregate, not a group, of participants who begin to meet together. Behavior in these early meetings is likely to reflect socially expected patterns of conversation and parallel participation, rather than interaction.

The meetings. Parents who attended the first meeting were married or formerly married parents of teenagers. They were white, of lower middle class status and had learned of the program from newspaper notices. Two social work field students were present as facilitators. They introduced themselves and discussed the purposes and potential of a parent group. Group purposes were described as providing an opportunity for mutual support and sharing of common problems, becoming better informed about foster care, and improving the ways natural parents are treated in the foster care system. The workers emphasized the importance of parents in foster care and the need for full parent involvement in all aspects of the project. An agreement on confidentiality was negotiated. A guest speaker then presented information on a subject of intense concern to parents, legal rights and court procedure.

Parent behavior in the first meeting reflected individual, rather than group-focused, participation but was not restrained social conversation. Parents were responsive to suggested group and project goals. They were very verbal in their questions and complaints to the guest. They sometimes interrupted one another to ask questions and poured out their experiences and feelings. At the meeting's end, parents expressed strong interest in continuing to have speakers and strong approval of a group forum for sharing common problems.

For at least the next two meetings, parents vented their hurt, frustration and anger. The workers, having once attempted unsuccessfully and inappropriately to have the parents "listen" more to the invited speaker, recognized and supported parent need to express feelings and share experiences with one another. During these initial meetings, all group facilitation, meeting arrangements and other decision-making was left to the workers. Parents began to interrelate more with one another starting with the third meeting. Complaints and challenges to the speakers began abating.

II. Group Formation Phase

Groups are in the process of formation once participants have some significance for each other, have common goals and some tasks, see the group as an entity, see themselves in the group, have set some expectations for behavior in the group, and have begun to establish a role system.

The meetings. The evidence for the group formation phase was clear by the sixth meeting, an evaluative and planning session. A core of 6-8 parents had been regularly attending. Led by the workers, these parents were highly involved in selecting specific issues on which the group could move to assist its members and other natural parents. They focused on the recruitment of additional members and the development of a brochure which would inform parents about the group and legal rights and processes. In a subsequent meeting, the group, with worker help, welcomed new parents, channeled hostility about county agency workers constructively into a list of suggestions to a receptive agency supervisor, and planned ahead for departure of the student workers.

In the eighth meeting, parents and workers evaluated group progress. Asked to describe themselves when they attended their first meeting, they used words or phrases such as "alone," "scared," "frustrated," "angry," "blamed," and "failure." They referred to early sessions as "crying in our beer" and pointed out clear group accomplishments by the eighth session: more understanding of the foster care system, a brochure for parents, and ability to take their concerns to appropriate persons or organizations. Clearly, members were pleased with their accomplishments and had moved from negative individual orientations to a positive group focus.

A change of student workers did not noticeably affect group functioning as anticipated. Transition planning and follow-through went smoothly. New and old staff met jointly with the parents group to reconfirm goals and wish the departing workers well.

There also was no subsequent evidence of Phase III, "Integration, Disintegration and/or Reintegration." According to Hartford, just when a group seems to form and settle down to its work, a radical change may occur which produces stronger integration, or disintegration and/or reintegration. This group appeared to move steadily from Phase II into Phase IV, "Group Functioning and Maintenance."

Group Composition by the End of the Group Formation Phase

Before describing the group work in Phase IV, it may be of interest to present a brief picture of group composition after 5 months of meetings. There were 17 parents who attended often, most of whom had teenagers in foster care; 8-10 of these parents attended regularly. Ages ranged from mid-30s to early 50s. There were four married couples and three married persons who attended without spouses. Five were divorced or separated women; one woman was never married. One couple was black; all other parents were white. Almost all parents were of lower middle class or upper lower class status.

A set of descriptions of typical group members follows. Since the project focus was not on parental functioning, there was no attempt to collect information about individual or family backgrounds.

> Katherine was divorced and in her early forties. A religious and softspoken woman, she had a teenage daughter in foster care. She felt left out of all planning for this child by the various youth and runaway services, juvenile court, social workers and foster families involved, until her daughter entered group home care. Group home services included contracting and planning with her as the parent. Katherine gave and received support in the group and was a responsible participant in many tasks.

> Linda was a married woman in her forties. Her teenage daughter was in foster home placement. Linda was angry with agency, juvenile court and juvenile services staffs, openly confronting these persons when she encountered them. Her interactions with the new foster parents were collaborative, partially as a result of her developing an altered view of foster care service and parent roles while in the group. She was active in group planning and participation.

> Tom was married, in his late forties, with a teenage daughter in foster care. He attended meetings after his wife had been attending for some time. Reserved in his initial meetings, he rapidly became an active, thoughtful participant and informal leader, particularly in maintaining the group's supportive emotional tone.

> Hal was married, in his early 50s. He and his wife attended every group meeting from the beginning. Angry and frustrated by his dealings with the county agency and courts regarding his teenage daughter, he continued to attempt to cooperate with them. He provided both support and leadership for social action throughout the group's experience.

> Sandra was in her 30s and separated from her husband for a number of years. Unable to work because of illness, she looked physically frail and tired. Her six children, all under age 12, were in foster placement. Sandra felt all her workers in the county social services system were against her and was unsure why her children were in care. She was uninformed about how foster care works. In the group she was a warm, if disorganized, participant and appreciative of group meetings.

Della was a single mother in her early 20s who attended irregularly. Her two children, ages 18 months and 3 years, were in foster homes in another county. She had recently lost her job and was living alone in a tiny apartment. Della had not heard from her worker nor received visits with her children in months, yet was hopeful that the juvenile court would return the children to her at the next scheduled hearing. She was a pleasant and dependent group member. She used the group's attention and concern to begin to get more information and make decisions about what actions she might take.

Phase IV, Group Functioning and Maintenance

In this phase the group is at work toward its goals. Group culture, norms, relationships and leadership patterns are stabilized. The group is important to its members; "we" is used often. The group worker often is able to take a less central role as the group assumes more responsibility for its maintenance and functioning.

The meetings. During the next eight meetings, the group worked enthusiastically on all aspects of the brochure from design and content to dissemination. The brochure was viewed as a service to other parents and as a means of recruiting new members. In addition, it strengthened the group bond and sense of identity. Members chose a name to be used on the brochure and had a logo designed. Simultaneously, they discussed how to build membership and what the group could offer parents. Workers, however, noted that their active facilitation continued to be needed.

Once the brochure was completed and distributed, the group discussed needs and goals. Less time was needed for core members to share stressful events, either because they had reached personal acceptance of their situations or because the original problem circumstances were stabilized. They continued their high interest in speakers and reaffirmed the wish to assist others. Irregular or occasional participants were less a part of the group. Some attended only when they were again in crisis. They received support and attention from group members at the meetings, but little extra-group follow-up. Some did not attend because they were in crisis. There was little active follow-up of these persons. Thus, new members, especially those who had young children in placement and were in crisis, often did not continue.

In the following eight to ten sessions, the group bond remained strong and activity level, high. Extra-meeting activities bolstered enthusiasm further. During this time, several members, working with the author, gave a well-received workshop for foster parents. Lapel buttons with the group logo were made and worn by members. Some members enrolled in a parent training course provided by an agency at the group's request. There also continued to be much extra-group contact and support among regular members.

Workers noted that most or all the many tasks of the group and project remained their responsibility, since members felt pressured by the other demands of their daily lives. Parents accepted some limited tasks, but were unwilling to take on major ongoing responsibilities. Leadership was not well developed, despite worker efforts to encourage leadership roles. Group facilitation by workers—particularly in clarifying issues, opinions, and decisions—continued to be needed.

By September 1977, about 25 group sessions had been held. In the next four months (7 sessions), some signs of disequilibrium began to show. This may have been a result of several interacting factors. One was the natural progression of some members toward termination. Another was the departure and replacement of one worker in September and one anticipated in December. These shifts resulted in some discontinuity in both worker functioning as a team and in level of group facilitation by the workers. A third factor was the realization that publicity efforts were not succeeding in increasing membership. Inappropriate behavior by some occasional participants at this time seemed to upset the group's equilibrium.

Phase III, Disintegration and/or Reintegration

The group during this period showed some of the characteristics of a bypassed earlier Phase III. Recontracting affirmed goals of developing membership and continuing efforts at change in how natural parents are perceived and treated. At the same time, workers noted an undercurrent of conflict and dissatisfaction. The group appeared hesitant to deal with member conflict in a straightforward manner. When an incident of some member insensitivity occurred, it was not dealt with by members or workers at the time. As a result, two members did not return, and others who continued were displeased with the outcome.

Most members continued to attend and to reaffirm goals. They anticipated the departure of one worker appropriately and were fully accepting of continuance with the remaining worker. Core members, now at a clearly different stage from new members, needed help in integrating new members into the group. When the group reconvened after winter holidays, it openly discussed its behavior and set norms for group behavior. This worked well and meetings continued on a more positive note. The later addition of a second student group worker delayed overall planning. When the group and staff met to review and recontract, several core members indicated their intention to leave the group.

Phase V, Termination

This marks the ending of a group. It encompasses three subphases: A. "pretermination," the acknowledgment of, and planning for, ending; B. "termination," the actual last group session, sometimes including an ending ceremony; and C. "post-termination," including reunion contact or follow-up services. Termination may occur for various reasons. The group may reach its planned time limit. The group may fail to coalesce. It may complete its task. Members may no longer need the group. It may experience the extensive loss of members and/or leaders, including the group worker(s). Some of these were factors in this group's ending.

The meetings. All parents and staff reaffirmed support for the group and project. The four core members who stated they no longer needed the group did not want the group to end, but felt they had "graduated." Their children were back home or reaching age of majority and leaving foster care. Four parents wished to continue. Two of them planned and suggested a modified group. A fifth, in crisis regarding a TPR hearing for her child, was unable to give attention to the decision-making.

Although members were available to continue in the group, a staffing reality resulted in termination of group meetings: no student workers would be available during the coming three summer months. The group planned to continue to meet until the current workers left. Together they reviewed accomplishments and tasks yet undone. While disappointed about the negligible increase in membership, they were pleased with community recognition and greatly satisfied with the mutual support and problem-sharing the group experience had offered. The group held a potluck party to honor its original members, thank its workers, and include agency and community "friends" of the two past years. After termination, parents maintained regular contact with one another.

Reflections on the parent group experience

Despite differences in context and parent group composition, the outcome of work with this natural parent group was consistent with the reports of group work with parents reviewed in Section I. These parents were participants in a project not focused on personal change and were somewhat older and of more stable socioeconomic status than most participants in other groups. Yet, there were many commonalities in their situations and their experiences with child welfare systems, in group processes and in effects of group participation. Parents reported feeling uninformed, isolated and negatively labeled and treated in foster care. They were active in meetings from the beginning and used the first several meetings to air their anger, hurt, guilt and concerns. The group's meaning for members was positive, yet its development was relatively slow. The convening and early group phases took relatively long periods of time; substantial levels of worker activity were necessary through the group's life. The need for continuing worker responsibility was partly due, of course, to the number and complexity of tasks required by the project. Of likely greater impact, however, were the debilitating effects on parents of continuing crises: the crises in their life situations, the crisis of loss of child(ren) and the crisis of dealing with the immense and intimidating foster care system as they experienced it. It is very promising that, given the ongoing demands on the energies of natural parents, group work can still have quite positive results. Parents became better informed about foster care, no longer felt isolated, contributed and received support and encouragement, and generally were able to interact with the foster care system more effectively. In addition, they formed a support network outside of the project activities. They demonstrated willingness and increasing ability to act as advocates on behalf of natural parents. As group members, the parents became able to effect some changes in how natural parents were treated and came to be viewed as resources by agency staff. These were evidence of the positive effects that group work can have on the providing agency, as well as on parent group participants.

Issues for Group Work with Natural Parents in Permanency Planning

Having looked conceptually at group work with parents in permanency planning and at an example of a group of natural parents, we will conclude with some issues and questions regarding the use of group work in permanency planning efforts. One set of issues includes ethical considerations relating to definitions of purpose and of client; the other set pertains to outcomes.

Permanency planning, while variously defined and implemented, always has the child in mind as beneficiary. Where family or parent needs conflict with the child's needs, the latter receive priority. Thus, the dilemma of group services in permanency planning is the potential for their misuse. The group member's rights to self-determination may be abridged by agency-imposed agendas (Levinson, 1973). The natural phases of group development may not "fit" the permanency planning timetable established by agency or legislative policy. More time may be needed for growth to occur, especially for seriously disadvantaged parents. The right to client confidentiality may conflict with an agency's wish to build a clear record against the parent(s) in court. These ethical dilemmas are avoidable. Group participation needs to be completely voluntary, so that rejection of the service modality does not carry threats or penalties of loss of children. Very clear and ethical contracting regarding group purposes and careful decisions about group composition in terms of purposes will help ensure that member needs and group goals are compatible. The nature and limits of confidentiality should be clarified within the agency and with potential group members.

Group work may have both successful and unsuccessful components for permanency planning outcomes. On the one hand, it may be viewed as less successful because it may take longer for observable positive changes in the behavior of some parents than current timelines would allow. Also, group work may not be used often enough or completely enough by parents in the lowest socioeconomic strata. Further, group work or any other treatment modality cannot and should not be expected to be a substitute for basic resources provision of shelter, food, clothing, and medical care.

On the other hand, group work may be seen as helping achieve more family stability. It provides a service otherwise rarely available to natural parents. It decreases parent isolation and strengthens self-esteem. It greatly increases parent understanding and acceptance of agency services. It can be designed differentially to help serve parents and their families at various points along the foster care continuum from needs identification through aftercare.

Group work is valuable to the agency as well. It produces improved worker attitudes toward natural parents and positive changes in worker-parent roles. It is an effective way of providing needed information and an excellent means of providing support to parents. It can produce innovations and improvements in agency training and informational resources. Where group services are used as part of permanency planning efforts, it will be very useful to document and report their explicit purposes, processes and outcomes in order to assess their impact on those efforts. Along with other needed research on permanency planning (Maluccio et al., 1980) such information could help provide direction for changes in service delivery. It will be helpful to learn what group work services with which natural parents at which points in the continuum of foster care will assist permanency planning efforts.

REFERENCE NOTE

1. This project is described in detail in Carbino, R. Developing a parent organization: New roles for parents of children in substitute care. In A. N. Maluccio and P. A. Sinanoglu (Eds.), *The Challenge of Partnership—Working with Parents of Children in Foster Care.* New York: Child Welfare League of America, 1981.

REFERENCES

American Public Welfare Association. *Potentials for Service Through Group Work in Public Welfare.* Chicago: American Public Welfare Association, 1962.

Avery, N. & Wayne, J. Group development and grief therapy for nonnurturing mothers. *Social Work with Groups,* 1978, *1,* 287-298.

Belluci, M. T. Group treatment of mothers in child protection cases. *Child Welfare,* 1972, *51,* 110-116.

Boyd, P. E. They can go home again! *Child Welfare,* 1979, *58,* 609-615.

Breton, M. Nurturing abused and abusive mothers: The hairdressing group. *Social Work with Groups,* 1979, *2,* 161-174.

Carbino, R. Developing a parent organization: New roles for parents of children in substitute care. In A. N. Maluccio and P. A. Sinanoglu (Eds.), *The Challenge of Partnership—Working with Parents of Children in Foster Care.* New York: Child Welfare League of America, 1981.

Carter, W. W. Group counseling for adolescent foster children. *Children,* 1968, *15,* 22-27.

Child Welfare League of America. *Group Method and Services in Child Welfare.* New York: Child Welfare League of America, 1963.

Child Welfare League of America's Statement on Foster Care Services. *Child Welfare,* 1979, *58,* 49-50.

Davoren, E. Working with abusive parents: A social worker's view. *Children Today,* 1975, *4,* 38-43.

Edinger, H. B. Reuniting children and parents through casework and group work. *Children,* 1970, *17,* 183-187.

Fanshel, D. *Computerized Information for Child Welfare: The availability and capacities of parents of children in foster care for service involvement.* New York: Columbia University School of Social Work, 1978.

Glasser, P. H. Methods in child welfare: Review and preview. *Group Methods and Services in Child Welfare.* New York: Child Welfare League of America, 1963, 5-11.

Hartford, M. E. *Groups in Social Work.* New York and London: Columbia Press, 1971.
Heiting, K. H. Involving parents in residential treatment of children. *Children,* 1971, *18,* 162-169.
Jones, B. M. A demonstration homemaker project. *Child Welfare,* 1964, *43,* 133-136.
Jones, M. A. Reducing foster care through services to families. *Children Today,* 1976, *5,* 7-10.
Kadushin, A. Substitute care: Foster-family care. *Child Welfare Services,* Third edition. New York: Macmillan Publishing Co., 1980, 313-412.
Kautz, E. S. Family services that obviate the need for child placement. *Child Welfare,* 1969, *48,* 289-295, 308.
Knitzer, J. & Allen, M. L. *Children Without Homes: An Examination of Public Responsibility.* Washington, D.C.: Children's Defense Fund, 1978.
Kruger, L., Moore, D., Schmidt, D., & Wiens, R. Group work with abusive parents. *Social Work,* 1979, *24,* 337-338.
Lahti, J., Green, K., Emlen, A., Zaomy, J., Clarkson, Q. O., Kuehnel, M., & Casciato, J. M. *A Follow-Up Study of the Oregon Project.* Portland, Oregon: Regional Institute for Human Services, Portland State University, 1978.
Lang, N. C. A comparative examination of therapeutic uses of groups in social work and in adjacent human service professions: Part II - The literature from 1969-1978. *Social Work with Groups,* 1979, *2,* 197-220.
Lee, J. A. & Park, D. N. A group approach to the depressed adolescent girl in foster care. *American Journal of Orthopsychiatry,* 1978, *48,* 516-527.
Levinson, H. M. Use and misuse of groups. *Social Work,* 1973, *18,* 66-73.
Ludlow, B. & Epstein, N. Groups for foster children. *Social Work,* 1972, 96-99.
Magnus, R. Parent involvement in residential treatment programs. *Children Today,* 1974, *3,* 25-27.
Maluccio, A. N., Fein, E., Hamilton, J., Klier, J. L., & Ward, D. Beyond permanency planning. *Child Welfare,* 1980, *59,* 515-530.
Maybanks, S. & Bryce, M. (Eds.) *Home-based Services for Children and Families.* Springfield, Ill.: Charles C. Thomas, 1979.
McFerran, J. Parents' groups in protective services. *Children,* 1958, *5,* 223-228.
Middleman, R. Returning group process to group work. *Social Work with Groups,* 1978, *1,* 11-26.
Montelius, M. Group services in public welfare agencies. In *Helping People in Groups.* Washington, D.C.: U.S. Department of Health, Education and Welfare, 1966, 1-16.
Murphy, D. A. A program for parents of children in foster family care. *Children Today,* 1976, *5,* 37-40.
Navarre, E., Glasser, P. H. and Costabile, J. An evaluation of group work practice with AFDC mothers. In P. Glasser, R. Sarri, & R. Vinter (Eds.), *Individual Change Through Small Groups.* New York: Free Press, 1974.
Peterson, J. B. & Sturgies, C. H. Group work with adolescents in a public foster care agency. In W. Schwartz & S. R. Zalpa (Eds.), *The Practice of Group Work.* New York: Columbia University Press, 1971, 122-143.
Pike, V. Permanent planning for foster children: The Oregon Project. *Children Today,* 1976, *5,* 22-25, 41.
Rose, S. Parent training in groups. *Group Therapy: A Behavioral Approach.* Englewood Cliffs, N.J.: Prentice-Hall, Inc., 1977, 166-181.
Rubenstein, H. After care, who cares? *Child Welfare,* 1967, *46,* 195-202.
Sauber, M. Preplacement situations of families: Data for planning services. *Child Welfare,* 1967, *46,* 443-449.
Shyne, A., Sherman, E. A., & Phillips, M. H. Filling a gap in child welfare research: Service for children in their own homes. *Child Welfare,* 1972, *51,* 562-573.
Shyne, A. W. & Schroeder, A. G. *National Study of Social Services to Children and Their Families.* Washington, D.C.: U.S. Department of Health, Education, and Welfare, Administration for Children, Youth, and Families, Children's Bureau, 1978.

Simmons, G., Gumpert, J., & Rothman, B. Natural parents as partner in child care placement. *Social Casework,* 1973, *54,* 224-232.

Stein, T. J., Early intervention in foster care. *Public Welfare,* 1976, *34,* 39-44.

Stein, T. J., Gambrill, E. D., & Wiltse, K. *Children in Foster Homes: Achieving Continuity of Care.* New York: Praeger, 1978.

Stone, H. D. *Reflections on Foster Care.* New York: Child Welfare League of America, 1969.

Sussman, M. B. The sociology and economics of foster care. In H. D. Stone (Ed.), *Foster Care in Question.* New York: Child Welfare League of America, 1970,183-191.

Torczyner, J. & Paré, A. The influence of environmental factors on foster care. *Social Service Review,* 1979, *53,* 358-477.

Vinter, R. D. An approach to group work practice. In R. D. Vinter (Ed.), *Readings in Group Work Practice.* Ann Arbor, Mich.: Campus Publishers, 1967, 1-7.

Watson, K. W. Preadolescent children in group discussions. *Children,* 1968, *15,* 65-70.

Weinbach, R. W., Edwards, M. J., & Levy, R. F. Innovations in group services to foster parents: A survey of agencies. *Children Today,* 1977, *6,* 18-20.

Wiltse, K. T. Decision-making needs in foster care. *Children Today,* 1976, *5,* 2-5, 43.

Winder, A., Ferrini, L., & Gaby, G. Group therapy with parents of children in a residential treatment center. *Child Welfare,* 1965, *44,* 266-271.

Planning with Parents: The Use of Groups in Residential Treatment

Carol Ackermann Mitchell

ABSTRACT. The relationship between parents of children in residential treatment and the agency is of concern to child welfare professionals who feel the burden of making permanent plans for the very troubled youngsters who "end up" in group facilities. This relationship is also of paramount concern to those parents who entrust their children to such care, and whose anxiety about sharing the care of their children often makes them appear unwilling or unable to participate in planning for them. The experience of one such program for latency boys suggests that outreach to families which includes various group services promoting parent-to-parent socializing, support and treatment can effectively involve parents in permanent planning efforts and can also bring changes in staff attitudes and agency practices.

Parents, group work, residential treatment, and placement planning have fit together awkwardly, if at all, in child welfare thinking. Parental guilt about *any* placement, professional notions of "saving" children from "bad" home environments, and milieu therapy approaches which emphasize regulation of outside (family) influences on the identified patient have conspired against active involvement of parents, both individually and in groups, in residential treatment. This lack of involvement, which is usually explained as parental "resistance" or "unworkability," complicates the crucial issue of permanency planning. This paper explores some problems and solutions to the issue of parental involvement in a residential treatment program.

The experiences of Walker Home and School in Needham, Massachusetts, suggest that parents of youngsters in residential treatment can be mobilized to involve themselves in planning for

---

At the time of this writing, Carol Ackermann Mitchell, MSW, was Clinical Associate at Walker Home and School, Needham, Massachusetts.

their children, and that the utilization of group work contributes to this parental involvement. Walker serves 34 residential and 18 day students, all boys ages 6 to 13, and offers a five-day program of on-grounds special education, a therapeutic milieu, weekly psychotherapy, and family work services. Treatment usually lasts 2 to 3 years and is funded by a combination of local education funds, state welfare monies, and private contributions. The 52 boys are from a broad range of socioeconomic backgrounds, and about 20% are minorities. Most boys eventually return to their families, although some go on to adoptive or foster homes, or to other treatment settings. Formal family group work has been a relatively recent addition in Walker's 20-year history (Trieschman et al., 1969).

Permanency Versus Residential Treatment?

Where does residential treatment fit in the spectrum of avenues to consider in permanency planning? The growing literature on the subject of "permanency planning" focuses on foster care as the temporary solution to be quickly replaced by a return to the natural family or by legal and social work efforts to effect an adoptive placement. Group care facilities are not mentioned. With the current jargon of "deinstitutionalization" in mind, long-term residential treatment of seriously disturbed youngsters can wrongly be viewed as antithetical to efforts to secure a permanent, healthy family environment for children. This view of group care as a "no man's land" where children languish while decisions are made by outside forces misunderstands the nature of residential treatment. Nor is residential care necessarily a first step toward the eventual dissolution of the natural family, an unspoken fear of many parents and a hidden assumption of some referring professionals.

As emphasized by Small (1979), Whittaker (1979), and others, the goal of residential treatment is to *enhance* family functioning by maintaining continuity of care via keeping the family as the locus of work from the beginning. If residential care is seen as a time-limited period of respite for child and family in which contact is not lost, the residential component can be part of the planned package of services whose goal is the strengthening of the natural family and the child's eventual full-time return. Residential programs are repeatedly reminded, by law and by progressive practice, that "[the child] is the *parents'* child and not the Home's" (Keith-Lucas and Sanford, 1977, pp. 249-250) and that "the parents have the right to know what is happening to his child, to participate in planning with and for the child, to make important decisions in the child's life.'' We are reminded by Sanford et al. that the residential program ''does not have the power to decide whether or not the parent should be involved. He is involved by the very fact that he exists . . . . Are we being ethical when we do not encourage the parent to participate responsibly? It is at the point of his active participation that we begin to help the parent understand his responsibility'' (Keith-Lucas and Sanford, 1977, p. 104).

Walker School's switch from a seven-day to a five-day program in 1973 served to enhance the family-treatment focus. When youngsters go home every weekend, the overriding planning issue is raised weekly: can this family and child benefit enough from the partial separation and the services offered that the outcome after 2-4 years will be going home full time?

Walker's experience has been that the result is not always reintegration into the natural family, although the great majority of Walker boys do return to their original home. For those families where the goal of returning home has been clear from intake for parents, referring and funding agencies, and the Walker treatment team, the years of residential and day care focus on strengthening the natural family. A second agenda is added when one or more of these parties (parents, referral source, or treatment center) are unsure of or in disagreement about what the long-term outcome should be. Then treatment to strengthen the family must go on simultaneously with consideration of other options, including adoption. Rather than a ''sequential approach'' of massive treatment efforts followed by discussion of other options, Epstein and Heymann (1967) advocate a ''selective approach'' in which all options are openly discussed from the beginning to avoid delays in planning. In effect, almost every facet of a residential facility's work with families can be seen as connected to the process of settling on and implementing a decision about a youngster's future that will link him firmly to those who will nurture and guide him/her to adulthood, i.e., permanency planning.

Encouraging Parent-to-Parent Contacts

Where, then, do group services to parents fit into a residential program whose goals are strengthening natural families and helping some families find alternative plans for their children? And how does the agency move from the first step, that parents should be actively connected with the institution staff, to the idea that parents should be actively connected with each other? As Small and Whittaker (1979) point out, there is "a pressing need to identify ways in which families can come together and be supportive of one another" (p. 11).

Like most seven-day residential programs, Walker in its early years tended to keep parents at bay, servicing them separately from their children, viewing them as responsible for the children's pathology—the "parents as perpetrators" stance taken by so much of psychoanalytic and developmental literature. Whittaker calls this the "family etiology hypothesis." The lack of involvement of parents other than on "visitors days" or at discharge did not make sense, however, if that meant returning an "improved" youngster to an "unchanged" home setting. So, at Walker and in residential and group treatment centers across the country, parents were increasingly welcomed as clients, as individuals with problems and needs of their own which, if treated, could make them more effective parents. For Walker, this trend, coupled with the switch to five-day treatment, led the families to look to staff who dealt with the boys, rather than to an outside service agency, for help with weekend behaviors they now faced.

The "parents as clients" stance meant that a full range of treatment services for parents became part of the child's treatment, dependent of course on staff skills and resources. The group modality was a logical addition, for groups had proven their worth in all types of treatment and parent guidance settings, given "the natural tendency of parents to discuss child-rearing problems with other parents" (Arnold et al., 1978, p. 114). While the parents of children in residence often have such complex, chronic, and difficult problems that the usefulness of group treatment might be questioned, at the same time they have an overwhelming need for such a modality. Often personally isolated and friendless, frequently so defeated by their sense of failure as people and as parents as to be unable to advocate for themselves and their children, sometimes feeling that they are the only parents in the world who have taken the drastic residential placement step, they are a client population most in need of the curative aspects of group treatment (Yalom, 1970). Yet groups for parents of emotionally or behaviorally disordered children have been slow to evolve. And residential programs, particularly those treating children from a wide geographic area, report substantial difficulties in starting therapy, support, or organizational groups among their parent-clients.

Walker School's small service area (Greater Boston) has been an important positive factor in the development of group services, although transportation is still a major roadblock to participation for some. At the present time, group gatherings are utilized from orientation day (intake) to graduation (discharge) in a variety of modes that range from all-school socials to traditional parent support groups. The relatively less "therapeutic" occasions are seen as part of "group services" when one realizes that it is often these informal occasions that promote enough parent-to-parent contact to lead to involvement in more formal group programs. The social events and happenstance contacts between parents have reduced staff anxieties about getting groups of parents together, and also led to suggestions from parents themselves that group services be offered.

The development of parent-to-parent contact was an inevitable part of inviting parents to the school, even in the early "keep parents at bay" days. Indeed, the first "parent group" formed naturally on visitors days, held every sixth Sunday, when the eight to twelve parents would come to see their boys, meet with the director, Dr. Trieschman, and gather informally for coffee. They would occasionally share rides to the school and even exchange phone numbers, developing an informal support network that suggested to Dr. Trieschman and other staff that promoting mutual support via groups would be a positive step.

Growing Parental Involvement via Groups

The first Walker parents group began in 1971, started by a social work student with the encouragement of the lone family worker on the staff at the time. The group was continued when the worker was hired on a part-time and then full-time basis, and as new members came and went, met weekly until 1974. Part of the rationale for the group was to cut back on the need for casework services, although the group turned out to require lots of energy from the leader and a co-leader who joined later. The mothers who participated were drawn from the caseloads of the two leaders, and were primarily single parents who needed support, a sense of not being alone, and help with management issues. The three to five mothers came in on Monday mornings, either in the cab with their boy or when they brought their son in themselves. They met for 1½ hours over coffee and donuts and discussed whatever topics they themselves brought up. The group ended when most of the mothers' sons left Walker, along with the two leaders. But the staff had seen the benefits of bringing parents together, and the idea of groups caught on.

The next two parent groups were organized in an effort to reach out to the parents who lived in Boston and did not have transportation to the school. One, co-led by a child care administrator and a social work student, tried in 1974 to bring together three to five inner city mothers to meet in their own homes, with transportation provided by the leaders. Keeping the group going took an enormous amount of energy, and attendance fluctuated and dropped off. After about six months the group was disbanded.

A second inner city mothers group, this one specifically for black parents, was organized in 1975 by a black clinician who drew from among the individual cases assigned to him. A major purpose was to help the women deal with the predominantly white suburban institution that was treating their children. During its second year, the group was co-led by a white female graduate student. Interestingly, the mothers' bitter disappointment with the men in their lives led to more conflict and distrust of the male co-leader than of his white colleague. The core group included six or seven women who needed much encouragement, reminder phone calls prior to the sessions, and transportation provided by the leaders in order to attend. A few meetings occurred at Walker, but they met most often in each others' homes, and once for a potluck meal at the female leader's home. The focus of the group eventually included mobilizing to deal with the Boston public school system most of their boys were returning to. The group ended when most members' sons left Walker in 1977.

The black mothers' concerns about entrusting their sons to a white treatment center in a white suburb were accepted as legitimate by the leaders, who eventually encouraged the group to make the first organized parent input into the Walker system. The culmination of the group's work was their request to present their views and suggestions to the Walker staff, which led to a talk by two mothers to a mandatory all-staff meeting. Administrative willingness to listen to the power of parental suggestions in areas such as haircuts, vocabulary, discipline styles in black families, and the hiring of more minority staff made the experience more than simply a chance to ventilate. Specific changes followed, including establishment of an affirmative action committee to recruit staff.

Perhaps without realizing the impact of this step, Walker had moved beyond the "parents as clients" attitude to begin seeing "parents as partners" in the treatment of their troubled youngsters. This came at a time when other forces were at work as well: the new special education law which in Massachusetts (and now nationwide) requires parental involvement and approval by signature of the drafting of special educational plans, the consumer movement, the parents' rights movement. An unexpected outcome of encouraging this and other parents groups, Walker found, was that parents gathering common strength to advocate for their children meant that Walker too would be an object of their criticisms and suggestions. The impact of the evolving "parents as partners" stance will be discussed later in this article.

Long-Term Support Groups

The impetus that created Walker's current long-term parent support groups came, not from the clinical staff, but from the residential child care workers. Long before there even was a clinical department, contacts between child care staff and parents, occurring via telephone and during parental visits, had been utilized creatively to teach management skills to parents. As described by Hammond (1973), the social worker who coordinated Walker's first such contacts, parents were encouraged to look to residence workers for specific help with topics such as tantrum management and the establishment of routines. The suggestion that this teaching of behavior management skills could also be effectively done in groups was made by child care supervisors and workers. This idea of using parent education groups dovetailed with Walker's presentation of itself as a "school" rather than a "treatment center."

The first such instructional parent group was established in the spring of 1977. Invitations to the 1½ hour, biweekly evening sessions were issued via letter to all families and announced the topic to be presented and discussed that week. Initial response was enthusiastic and for the first few meetings attendance was high (10-12 parents out of 50 families). Some transportation was provided for inner city parents. However, attendance quickly fell off, and the organizers attributed the decline to the method of group leadership chosen. For each session, two different child care workers, or a child care worker and a clinician, volunteered to address a specific topic, but the leadership changed each time. The lack of continuity and carryover must have been disconcerting to the participants. However, the basic idea of a management/parent guidance group appeared sound.

The present form of Walker's biweekly, evening support group was launched in the fall of 1977 with two consistent staff leaders, one an experienced child care worker and one a clinical associate. All parents were invited to join, and attendance was voluntary. The group was and still is an adjunctive treatment and does not replace the direct family work service offered by the clinical staff. The group format for the first 2½ years continued to be that of a parent-education model, with leaders or guest speaker preparing brief talks to be followed by group discussion and sharing. Reminder letters and sometimes phone calls were utilized, and transportation from a nearby subway station was offered to urban parents.

Transportation problems for the inner city parents, coupled with marked socioeconomic and personal differences, led to a split in the Needham-based group. A few former members of the black mothers group were also interested. However, it was not until the fall of 1978 that two staff members were able to add the Boston group to their workload. The new leaders were a teacher interested in family work and a social work graduate student. The group used space, first at a school for social work, and for the last two years, in a church in a central and racially neutral area of the city.

The two parent support groups have become an established part of Walker's program. Participation continues to be elective and in addition to regular family work services, although in some cases the frequency of the individual family sessions has been reduced. When changes in group leadership have occurred, efforts have been made to keep one male and one female leader, if possible from different departments within the agency, i.e., clinical and child care. The model now used falls somewhere between the group guidance and group therapy approaches (see Arnold et al., 1978), drawing features from each. Membership is open-ended, with new parents joining and others dropping out, and the groups lack the firm commitment required in traditional group therapy. Both groups have at times utilized an instructional model with emphasis on giving information and advice. Yet both groups have evolved toward extensive sharing of personal feelings and experiences, and members talk about their own problems and pasts, look at the group process, and seem to feel a commitment to each other to attend regularly.

Despite similarities, the two groups have distinct differences in membership and style. From the beginning the urban group was composed of poor, single mothers, most black, one a white woman from anti-black South Boston. Personal disclosure and discussion of their own issues were accepted from the beginning as legitimate.

Rather than the lecture format of the suburban group, the Boston group began meetings with "what's on top," and personal issues as well as behavior management and long-range planning for their sons were recurrent topics. Leaders had to expend much energy in phone calls and providing transportation to keep the group attendance up to three to four members per week. The intensity and usefulness of the sessions for those who did come, particularly for those anticipating their youngsters' graduation from Walker, had to be weighed against flagging attendance and the leaders' sense of "burnout." The original co-leaders left Walker after two years, and new co-leaders have revived the group by adding parents from the new intake group for an average attendance of four to five women.

The suburban group, now in its fourth year, originally consisted of six to ten parents, couples and formerly marrieds, who were able to provide their own transportation to the school. This self-selection led to an all-white group of working class and some middle class parents who at first were more interested in an educational approach. Meetings began with a talk requested by members and delivered by a leader. Topics included temper tantrums, lying, stealing, sibling rivalry, the basics of Parent Effectiveness Training, and so on. On one occasion a single mother spoke about her experiences. Discussion following the talk usually was child-focused, included much advice-giving between parents, and rarely touched marital or interpersonal concerns. After 2½ years of such meetings the group moved more toward a therapy model by discarding the topical format. Parents were surprised to find they did "have things to talk about" without it, and soon the group focused more on their own parenting troubles. To this new openness was soon added an acknowledgment of themselves as people apart from their children, with their own needs, issues and problems. This has been accompanied by increased group cohesion and more regular attendance. For the first time, two "alumni" families have elected to remain part of the group after their sons left Walker.

The permanency planning issue has been a more overt issue for some parents in the Needham group who are considering options other than the child's return to the family upon graduation. Two families have their sons already in partial foster care on weekends and are awaiting the location of long-term alternative families. Another couple periodically requests such relief care in panic, though it was rarely implemented, and a fourth mother has temporarily surrendered the care of her son to his father. One of these couples dropped out of the group for a number of months while the decision for foster care was being made, apparently feeling that the group would be angry at them for failing to improve their parenting in the face of an onslaught of "good advice" from the group. They returned with support and encouragement from the leader and were able to tell the group about the foster care plan. Two others voiced concerns about whether they were still entitled to attend the group since they were not to be the primary caretaking parents. One mother made the difficult decision to surrender her boy for adoption and relied heavily on group support to deal with her disapproving family and her own guilt. Disclosure of these alternative plans to the group has been met with support rather than rejection, and hopefully this support will continue to sustain the families once the planned foster and adoptive placements are made.

Short-Term Groups

Out of the long-term groups came suggestions for easing the transition for families entering and leaving Walker. Coupled with staff interest in improving intake and discharge procedures, these suggestions resulted in three types of short-term groups: a single session Orientation Day meeting, a four to five session weekly evening orientation group series for new parents, and a one or two session information and planning seminar for parents of graduates.

Since new students enter the school on one of two days (beginning of the summer, Labor Day), efforts to orient the new families as a group could be facilitated. The day before the boys were to move into residence, they and their parents could be invited as a group to receive information previously given individually via the intake workers. The first Orientation Day, in June 1977, included talks by clinical, education, and child care staff for the parents, a slide show for the boys, and a staff-family picnic. Though a success, this first format failed to promote much interaction among the dozen or so parents attending.

The tone of subsequent Orientation Days was improved by participation of current Walker parents as "resource parents." The first year's resource parents were group members who suggested that it would have helped them as "new" parents to have been able to talk to an "old" experienced parent. With some trepidation, staff invited six or seven resource parents to participate in the 90-minute parent-staff information and question session. The resource parents were asked to say whatever they thought new parents needed to hear. They also could remain quiet at the meeting and just be available to chat with new parents at the picnic. What ensued was most moving, for staff, resource parents, and new parents alike. Without prompting, the resource parents spoke about how awful it has been to place their boy in residence, how hard it was to trust staff initially, about their criticisms of the school, and about the progress they had seen. A few mentioned the parent groups in an effort to recruit new members. Their mere presence seemed to instill hope, and "imprinted" on new parents a view of the place and its services that staff could never have communicated. Mingling between parents at the picnic was more relaxed and gave new parents a chance to speak privately to the resource parents.

The use of resource parents has continued, with an effort made to ask a mix of parents from different backgrounds and with varied speaking abilities, rather than those most articulate or positive about the program. The response to being asked is almost universally, "what do *I* have to offer?" The ego-enhancement and boost to the self-esteem of individual parents was an important, if unexpected, by-product of the program. Those who felt like failures as parents saw that they had something valuable to give their peers and that staff respected what they could offer. A recent questionnaire on parent services confirmed the value of the Orientation Day program.

The short-term evening new parent orientation group is offered in addition to the Orientation Day informational meeting to continue extra support to the families through the child's first weeks at Walker. Instead of being invited directly into the ongoing support groups, new parents are offered a series of guest speakers to answer questions about the program and are also encouraged to share their feelings and reactions to the separation of placement. These groups are crucial in reassuring parents that they continue to be an important part of their child's life and that the school is not attempting to usurp their role as parents. Although voluntary when first offered in 1977, the four to five weekly sessions are now presented to new parents as a mandatory part of the intake process. Perhaps because of its time-limited contract, most new parents do attend the orientation group, even those who are not interested in the ongoing support groups.

The third type of short-term group has been less successful. The one or two session termination or "graduation" groups offered to families as their boys leave Walker have been sparsely attended. The format has been didactic, with an emphasis on dealing with public schools, private day programs, and funding agencies. The second session is a visit from a former Walker parent who can share "what life is like after Walker." Perhaps low attendance is due to holding the meetings so late in the year when decisions and anxieties may have already been discussed. Perhaps those parents who want to discuss transition issues do so in the support groups. Or perhaps at a time when families are disconnecting from the agency there is little energy available to invest in yet another talking group.

Impact of Groups on the Agency

The utilization of various types of parent groups at Walker has coincided with a shift in attitude toward families and the role they play in effective residential treatment of their children. Interest in treating client-parents in groups was followed by growing awareness that parents are partners as well, both in planning for their own particular children and in advocating for improved agency services. Not all Walker parents are active in non-client roles, and some parents do resist the more familiar client role. Yet, groups have played a key role in helping individual parents feel more secure in offering feedback and suggestions, and are often the vehicle for such communications.

The impact on the agency has been substantial. Administrators have been willing to implement specific parent suggestions: to publish a parent newsletter, to have school photos taken of the boys, to make changes in the graduation program and cookout. There is also an effort to enlist parent feedback ahead of time: rewriting the parent handbook, drafting a parent-agency placement agreement, changing the summer calendar affecting boys' vacation time at home. Suggestions from a recent three-page questionnaire to which about half of the parents responded are still being analyzed. And more receptive staff attitudes have coincided with the willingness of some parents to give back more directly: helping coordinate the annual graduation cookout which is now a potluck meal, serving as resource parents, offering individually to help out in clubs or in classes, to talk about their occupations or make "goodies" for bake sales. This volunteerism has not led, as staff had hoped, to a willingness to serve on agency committees or help with the newsletter or to the formation of a real parent-staff organization. Nor is the staff ready to open to scrutiny the everyday policies and functioning of the school in a way that would give parents real power over day-to-day decisions.

The greatest impact of the changing role of parents continues to be attitudinal. Teachers and child care workers feel freer to interact directly with families, rather than through the social workers, in order to address jointly the academic and behavior problems of the boys. Parent attendance at clinical conferences in which long-term recommendations are formulated was unheard of a few years ago; now such participation is allowed and invited by the treatment teams. The tension over "whose kids are they" that can easily develop between staff and parents is minimized by closer, more positive contacts. And the realization that both parents and surrogate parents (the staff) encounter the same problems in dealing with the child leads to more relaxed sharing about how to address those problems. Permanency planning is enhanced when the need to "rescue" kids gives way to an understanding on the part of all staff of the problems the parents are trying to overcome in coping with their children.

Impact on Families

It is difficult to measure the breadth of the impact that changes in services offered and in staff attitudes have on the parents Walker serves. The recent parent questionnaire suggests that, for those responding, the diverse contacts with staff are for the most part seen as helpful, and that contacts such as being invited to a residence dinner or science fair, or assistance with cab problems, or parent-teacher conferences, are valued just as much by some parents as the more traditional individual and group clinical services. Presumably the non-responding parents might take a more critical view. But the growing presence of families and extended families at social and program events and the increased clinical involvement with grandparents, both parents in divorced families and with siblings, all point to the conclusion that families feel more welcome at Walker than they used to. One also senses that the increased contact helps some parents see staff as people, too, making parents sympathetic to staff frustrations in dealing with the children and minimizing the possibility of youngsters manipulating parents against the staff.

Applications in Other Settings

How can other agencies apply what Walker has learned from its group experiences to enhance their own permanency planning endeavors? Most residential programs say they would like to provide group services and many have already attempted to do so, sometimes with little success. The first lesson Walker learned was that the provision involved commitment on an administrative level as well as the enthusiastic interest of the clinicians and child care staff who would actually run the groups. This agency commitment meant a willingness to allocate staff time and resources to an outreach which would show little obvious "payback" for some time. With this population it would be a mistake to assume low attendance meant that the parents who did attend got little from the experience. To assess results means asking the parents, not just the staff, to evaluate the value of the group program.

Implementing the decision to organize parent groups takes lots of effort. Walker found it helpful to have co-leaders and to pick them from two different roles within the agency (i.e., clinical and child care). It was also useful to have the leaders start recruiting members from among those with whom they *already* had regular and positive contact. Once connected to a few interested parents, this core group could be used for ideas and outreach to others. Having other parents already involved makes it easier for the reluctant parents or those who do not already know the leaders to get involved. Walker also utilized whatever occasions brought parents together (i.e., PTAs, orientations, science fairs, etc.) to encourage parent-to-parent interaction and sometimes to openly recruit group members. Leaders also had to see as part of their job helping prospective members with transportation, including arranging car pools or driving members themselves. Treatment centers whose population lives too far away may want to consider locating the group in another city near a cluster of families, with the leaders doing the most travelling. Another alternative would be to schedule them on visitors' days at the center. A particularly important support to Walker's group leaders was regular group supervision of their work in an effort to minimize discouragement and burnout.

Issues which need to be addressed in any such group include frequency of meetings, how didactic versus problem-oriented the content will be, how confidentiality will be handled among members and between the staff leaders and other center staff working with the families, and whether new members can join or others drop out at any time in the life of the group.

Conclusion

Only in an atmosphere of cooperation and mutual respect can productive planning for children occur. Both for the families growing stronger in anticipation of their child's return from residential treatment, and for those who need the strength to let go and allow their child to be raised by others, an approach which encourages parental partnership in permanent planning is essential. As Keith-Lucas (1977, p. 250) suggests, "only in such an atmosphere of mutual respect and common action does the state (or the agency) have the right to judge a parent on the way in which he exercises his rights and fulfills his responsibilities while the child is in his care. One cannot expect a parent to act responsibly if he is treated like trash." To engage the strengths and best ego functioning of our parent-clients in making permanent plans for their children, we must also respect and welcome them as partners and as people.

REFERENCES

Arnold, L. Eugene, Row, Marjorie, & Tolbert, Herman A. Parents Groups. In L. Eugene Arnold (Ed.), *Helping Parents Help Their Children,* New York: Brunner/Mazel, Inc., 1978, 114-125.

Epstein, Laura, & Heymann, Irmgard. Some Decisive Processes in Adoption Planning for Older Children. *Child Welfare,* Jan. 1967, 5-9, 46.

Hammond, John W. II. Child Care Workers as Helpers to Parents. *Child Care Quarterly,* 1973, *2*(4), 282-284.

Keith-Lucas, Alan & Sanford, Clifford W. (Eds.) *Group Child Care as a Family Service.* Chapel Hill, N.C.: University of North Carolina Press, 1977.

Small, Richard W., & Whittaker, James K. Residential Group Care and Home-Based Care: Toward a Continuity of Family Service. In M. Bryce & S. Maybanks (Eds.), *Home-Based Services for Children: Policy, Practice and Research.* Springfield, Ill.: Charles C. Thomas, 1979.

Trieschman, Albert E., Whittaker, James K., & Brendtro, Larry K. *The Other 23 Hours: Child Care Work in a Therapeutic Milieu.* Chicago: Aldine, 1969.

Whittaker, James K. *Caring for Troubled Children.* San Francisco: Jossey-Bass, Inc., 1979.

Yalom, Irvin D. *The Theory and Practice of Group Psychotherapy.* New York: Basic Books, 1970.

A Group Work Approach to Post-Surrender Treatment of Unwed Mothers

William Chiaradonna

ABSTRACT. This paper examines the development and use of a short-term group work approach to providing treatment to women who have surrendered a child for adoption. The clients' experiences during pregnancy, after the birth of their child, and following their surrender are discussed in the context of the group process. Further, an attempt is made to identify the major issues facing these clients and to suggest ways in which group treatment can help them deal with the underlying problems while supporting their adjustment to a most difficult life crisis.

Introduction

There has been a continual decrease in the number of women who surrender their babies for adoption. Paradoxically, however, the need for extended service to these clients is more urgent now than ever. A recent study comparing the characteristics of unmarried mothers who kept their babies with those who surrendered them for adoption points out that in the 1950s and early 1960s a white unmarried woman who kept her baby was deviating from accepted social norms (Grow, 1979). The current change in attitudes towards sex, marriage, and the traditional two-parent family, however, has altered that situation. Today, the number of single-parent families is on the increase, and the white mother who keeps her baby is more generally accepted in today's society.

As a direct consequence of the increased trend towards single parenthood, women who surrender their children for adoption now constitute a distinct minority. It is not unusual for these women to report that they have never known anyone who has surrendered her

William Chiaradonna, MSW, is the Group Service Coordinator at Charitable Bureau of Boston.

baby and that as a result, they feel totally isolated. Furthermore, they often report feeling that they are looked down upon because of their decision. In some cases they are even chastised or ridiculed by family and peers. The tables seem to have been turned. It is now women who choose adoption who deviate from the norm and are in need of special help if they are to cope adequately with the unique set of problems confronting them.

A Theoretical Perspective

In her book, *Unwanted Pregnancy and Counseling,* Juliet Cheetham (1977) explores the effects of psychological factors and how they influence women during and after their pregnancy. Cheetham points out that during the last trimester of pregnancy, many women experience a period of restlessness, anxiety, and, in some cases, panic as they come closer to the point at which their fantasies will encounter the reality of the infant and of themselves as a mother. This is a time when a woman becomes very much aware of the feelings connected with being a woman and a mother which reawakens her feelings about her own childhood and her own mother. It also revives the memories of forgotten conflicts and problems of those earlier times. Pregnancy often brings with it the fear of a change in a young woman's relationship with the father of her unborn child and the fear of abandonment by him. Under these circumstances, if her family does not provide the understanding and support that she needs, her fear of abandonment is compounded, and her concerns over the responsibilities she must face may be overwhelming. She must re-examine her roles and, often times, she is forced to abandon the more comfortable and familiar roles and relationships for new ones that are less familiar. The pregnant teenager must begin to anticipate her responsibilities as a mother, relying heavily on her own experiences with her mother and father to provide the basis on which to decide whether or not she possesses the resources and confidence that will enable her to meet the needs of her baby, while at the same time fulfilling her own needs. Her self-assessment in this regard obviously has far-reaching implications for her decision to surrender or keep her child.

A study by Carol Nettleton (1972) of unmarried mothers who made their decision to either keep or surrender their child provides some important data on the factors that influence a woman's decision. The women who surrendered listed their feeling that their baby needed two parents as the major factor that influenced their decision. They listed financial issues as the second most important concern and elaborated on their answers by noting their desire to finish school and their inability to provide for their child as well as an adoptive couple might be able to. Other issues that were reported as having affected the decision of those who surrendered were their age and unresolved feelings about the alleged father.

The opinion of the unmarried mother's family seemed to be another important factor. The women who kept their babies indicated that their family's opinion was the major factor influencing their decision. They felt that their parents supported their plan, offered them a place to live and acted in the role of involved grandparents. The women who surrendered, however, felt that the opinion of their parents influenced their decision less than many other factors. Ironically, many of these same women noted that their parents had indicated a strong preference in favor of surrendering. In addition, their parents pointed out that babies need two parents, the very same issue that the women felt influenced them most. One might speculate that parental feelings and attitudes might have had a stronger influence on the decision-making process than the women who surrendered were consciously aware of or able to admit.

The Nettleton study also goes on to discuss the areas of adjustment for unmarried mothers following their decision regarding their baby. The areas of adjustment which the women were asked to rank as being more or less difficult were:

1 - returning to the community
2 - family's attitudes towards her
3 - returning to school and/or work
4 - accepting the decision with regard to baby
5 - dating
6 - accepting oneself
7 - other

Among those who had surrendered, the most difficult area of adjustment was "learning to live with one's decision." A close second was "accepting oneself." The report pointed out the women's feelings of emptiness and wonderment regarding the welfare of the child. These concerns seem to be noted elsewhere in the literature as well (Burgess, 1975; Cheetham, 1977). The women also expressed a need to suffer in some way, and they experienced a sense of guilt if they were not suffering. They seem to have badly damaged self-concepts, especially in terms of their sexuality and their idea of themselves as trustworthy individuals. Finally, these women emphasized the problem they faced in regaining the trust and respect of family members.

The writer's own experience indicates that in addition to, but interwoven with, these concerns about trust and respect are feelings of anger and bitterness towards family members and others for what is perceived as their lack of support and failure to acknowledge what these women have been through. These feelings proved not only to be of major importance in post-surrender group treatment, but they were also the key factors in successfully engaging these clients in treatment. It was the anger and frustration that the women felt over what had happened that finally brought them to the post-surrender group.

Why Group Work?

Agencies have long recognized the need for post-surrender services for women who have surrendered their babies for adoption. The fact is, however, that many clients flee from ongoing casework treatment after they have legally surrendered. Often they express the need to put the experience behind them and to get on with their lives. A closer look reveals that such clients may have so much difficulty dealing with their own emotional distress that they project their guilt onto the agency or, more specifically, the caseworker, who then becomes the scapegoat for their displaced anger. As a result, workers find that their attempts to provide post-surrender casework services are met with a great deal of hostility and resistance.

The decision of the Catholic Charitable Bureau of Boston to consider an alternative approach to servicing this client population came from requests made by clients themselves. After surrendering their babies, some of these women felt that neither family, friends, nor professionals really understood what they had been through. They felt their experience was unique and that only other women who had surrendered a baby for adoption could understand how they were feeling. As a result, a few of these women suggested that it would be helpful to them to have an opportunity to talk with other women who had been through a similar experience. In response to their requests, the agency began to explore the possibility of developing a group work approach to post-surrender treatment.

A look at the literature reveals a variety of services currently available to the unmarried mother. Although group work approaches are not uncommon, the groups usually focus on the question of whether or not to surrender the baby or deal with parenting issues for those who keep their babies. Mention of post-surrender groups is rare. Clearly there is a need to consider how groups can be useful to women who make up the post-surrender population.

Roulet (1969) suggests that group therapy techniques open certain avenues that might not be possible to enter through individual psychotherapy. In particular, group work enables the members to exchange ideas and feelings among themselves and to dilute as necessary the relationship with the therapist. Nettleton (1972) suggests that by the fourth month after the surrender, the majority of these women will have continued or returned to some type of dating relationship and will be facing encounters in which they feel particularly vulnerable and/or which promote hurt regarding unresolved feelings of sexuality. She suggests that the use of the group can help these women answer the questions: "What am I saying about myself?", "What are my emotional needs?", "How can I effectively meet them in a less hurtful manner to myself and others?" The group helps to improve communication skills and provides for emotional support by one's peers, especially as the women become active again in male/female relationships.

There are many aspects of group therapy that seem tailor-made for post-surrender treatment. In outlining the curative factors in group therapy, Yalom (1975) offers a detailed account of various group phenomena which can contribute to the treatment of the post-surrender client. The group often provides a setting in which there is an improved opportunity for the installation of hope, a factor which is so important to help sustain the client in treatment and allow her to see the group as having potential to be of help to her. The client who has given up her child for adoption comes to the group and has the opportunity to see how other group members negotiate problems that are similar to her own. Some of them have faced these problems and are already coping more successfully, while others may be facing these problems less successfully themselves. In the first case, a client may gain hope that the problem can be dealt with effectively, and in the second she can gain hope through the realization of the progress she has already made as compared to others in the group. There is also the hope that one will be better understood and more likely to be helped by a group of people who have shared many of these problems.

Clients of many types enter treatment, whether individual or group, with the feeling that they are the only people in the world who feel so badly about themselves, that their problem would be totally unacceptable or frightening to others, or that they are having an inappropriately difficult time dealing with their situation. This is particularly true of clients in the post-surrender population. These women consistently report experiencing what they perceive as insensitivity and denial on the part of friends and relatives. Unfortunately, whether these feelings are legitimate responses to actual experiences or represent a projection of their own unresolved ambivalence, they cause the unwed mother to cut herself off from those with whom she might have discussed her experiences and shared her feelings. Furthermore, their sense of worthlessness and loneliness seems to be constantly reinforced by such feelings. Being in the group and sharing with and listening to others who have had similar feelings about their experiences helps to universalize their difficulties, and overcoming their sense of isolation aids them in dealing with their problems. They are no longer cut off from "everyone else." They have found a point of re-entry into society. The group offers an opportunity to talk about all of those issues that have made these women feel unworthy and have led them to question their roles and identity. It allows them to undergo experiences in an environment where they are unlikely to be exposed to the sort of condemnation by others which they have come to expect.

The group can also provide the client with the experience of giving to and receiving from others in the group. Some clients, especially in the early stages of the group's life, can give very little of themselves. For them, and for the group as a whole, the emotional gains that are achieved through observing the give and take between others should not be overlooked. The importance of receiving support, reassurance, suggestions, or insight from others in the group who are able to give more easily cannot be devalued, nor can the importance of groups in helping members to develop socializing techniques and in offering the benefits of role modeling and imitative behavior be underestimated.

Re-entering relationships with family, friends, or co-workers and beginning to gain confidence and feel better about oneself are very important matters for the post-surrender client. While these clients already have many skills in interpersonal relations, they may need an opportunity to test out their expectations and fantasies in a safe setting. They may have to improve or sharpen their skills in order to feel comfortable in dealing with the insensitivity and cruelty that they anticipate or experience in their day-to-day routine. The experience of negotiating with others and testing defenses in the group helps prepare the client for what she encounters outside the group. In addition, the group provides a variety of role models that the client can choose to imitate collectively or differently. Some of what she imitates may be permanently incorporated into her own behavior, but even that which she adopts temporarily may free her to deal with situations more comfortably.

Group Formation

Recruiting women for the group was a difficult task. The first obstacle was the reluctance of caseworkers to refer their clients. Many workers had been the recipients of clients' displaced anger following the surrender. Others experienced a great deal of resistance from clients who wanted to avoid post-surrender counseling. As a consequence, workers were sometimes hesitant about contacting clients who had terminated prematurely or fled the agency in anger. The second problem was the resistance of the women who were referred. Many clients who were invited to participate in the group declined saying that they had already worked out their problems and had adjusted to their situation. This was especially true of women who had surrendered six months to a year prior to our outreach efforts. Others who had surrendered just prior to the start of the group felt they were too upset to participate. Most of the women who became members of the group had already dealt with the initial grief reactions to the loss of their child. Even though some came to the group with ambivalence or regret about their decisions, most clients expressed a need for support and understanding and help with readjustment problems.

In composing groups at the Catholic Charitable Bureau of Boston, the issue of time was found to be an important consideration, as it relates to where the client is in regard to adjusting to her decision, returning to the community, and dealing with the problems she encounters. A mixture of women who are at different stages of readjustment appears to be helpful. Regardless of where the client is along this continuum, she can benefit from the experiences of others. They serve as a source of hope. They afford her an opportunity to compare her own experience and progress with those of her peers. The actions and comments of others in the group create a variety of situations which she can look at subjectively, while working through the effect that they have on her.

The two groups were composed of women ranging in age from their mid-teens to their mid-twenties. There were six women in the first group and three in the second. While both groups were productive and worthwhile, the larger group was more active, allowed for a broader range of experiences, and provided a greater exchange of problems, feelings, and suggestions among the group members. The wide age range created only minor problems since the groups were very narrowly focused and the women shared some important similar experiences regardless of their ages. The group workers also helped to minimize potential problems by recognizing and acknowledging differences and using them to contrast and compare situations and experiences.

It is important to note that because of the very small population from which to draw referrals and the limited time frame during which these clients can realistically be engaged in post-surrender treatment, the screening and selection process is very limited and group composition may have to be compromised if there is to be any group at all.

The Group Experience

A great deal of planning went into making the groups as attractive as possible to the target population. At the outset, it was decided that the groups should be short term to accommodate clients who had already expressed feelings that they didn't want treatment prolonged indefinitely, which they anticipated might be the situation in individual treatment. If the group decided that they needed more time to deal with unresolved issues, the contract could be renegotiated and the group extended or reorganized.

The groups, led by co-therapists, met for ten sessions of one and a half hours. They were held during the dinner hour, sandwiches and beverages being provided by the agency. As many of these clients worked in the metropolitan area, an early evening "dinner meeting" allowed them to come directly to the group from work, thus eliminating the extra time, expense, and inconvenience of commuting home for dinner and returning to the group later in the evening. This format also provided a more relaxed setting and seemed to relieve some of the anxiety that is so common among clients in more traditional group psychotherapy. Overall, this approach strongly reinforced the supportive nature of the group and heightened the familial frame of reference.

The group can offer clients a valuable opportunity to work on issues that are familial in origin. The group setting is much more effective in this regard than individual therapy, because of the similarities between the group and the family and the multiple transference that develops. The structure of the group and the interaction among the participants often resemble the configuration and dynamics of the family. The use of co-therapists, especially when they are male and female, further reinforces these similarities by providing symbolic parents. Finally, serving food and recreating a setting not unlike the family dinner table adds a nurturant quality to the group. Even though there are obviously wide disparities between the group and the family, the client's transference allows the similarities to emerge. This revives thoughts and feelings about family issues and promotes discussion of related problems.

During the ten sessions, a wide range of topics were discussed. Some of the central themes were:

1. Experiences during pregnancy
   a. hiding pregnancy
   b. isolation and loneliness
   c. parental attitude and their influence
   d. issues of autonomy vs. dependency
2. Reactions to the decision and subsequent surrender
3. Issues of grief and loss
4. Self-image and readjustment

The Early Sessions

Because of the limited time frame that was established for the group, the early sessions became crucial to the workers' efforts to build cohesion and trust among the members. Garland, Jones, and Kolodny (1973) refer to the first stage of group development as the "Pre-affiliation Stage." They define it as an "approach and avoidance" period during which members desire to become involved and get acquainted with one another while maintaining a safe distance, protecting themselves from the awkwardness and discomfort they anticipate. During the early sessions of the post-placement groups, the workers supported mutual exploration, but allowed the group members to maintain distance and progress at their own pace.

Although several sessions passed before the women began to become comfortable with each other, this approach successfully facilitated group cohesion and promoted trust.

The women used the early sessions quite appropriately. As discussions developed, the group focused on their experiences during pregnancy, an area which proved to be a safe topic of conversation. The incidents and events described by the clients were experiences that they had long since become comfortable with. By staying clear of more emotionally charged issues, they established a safe environment in which to get acquainted. The conversation allowed each woman to be a participant and an observer, testing her own ability and scrutinizing the actions and reactions of others.

Experiences during Pregnancy

> The first session began with a lot of small talk. After everyone had helped themselves to the food that had been provided, the leaders introduced themselves and explained why they had decided to organize a post-surrender group. They then asked the women to introduce themselves and tell each other a little bit about themselves and their experiences.
>
> Nancy began by telling the group that her baby was born last winter. She had a baby girl that weighed about ten pounds. With this Betty commented that she thought her baby was big at six pounds. Jane indicated that her baby was also ten pounds at birth. Nancy continued, telling the group that she had stayed at home throughout her pregnancy.
>
> Jane interrupted, saying that she stayed at a maternity home. She said she really liked being there because there were other girls in the same situation to talk to. At times, she admitted, it was a little boring, but they had groups like this one that she enjoyed participating in. In order to explain her lengthy absence from home, her family had developed an elaborate story in which she was supposed to have gone to work at a summer camp, had an accident on the way home, and had to stay in the hospital.
>
> Betty, somewhat nervously smiling and twisting her head, said her situation was really kind of different. She was living in Boston and her parents lived in Philadelphia so she never had to tell them. She said she was living with her sister who suspected she was pregnant but wasn't sure. During a visit to

her parent's home, however, her sister gained the support of two other siblings and they confronted her. Betty confirmed their suspicions, but to the best of her knowledge, no one ever told her parents and they still don't know.

Jane said she had gone to the maternity home partly to keep her pregnancy from her younger brother, but she doesn't think she was successful. He never came right out and asked her, but she thinks he knows.

Nancy, who had listened quietly up to this point, said she never tried to hide her pregnancy. She stayed home and did the things she usually did. Unfortunately, however, she learned quickly who her friends were. A lot of people tried to give unsolicited advice and force their values and opinions on her.

Betty said part of her problem was that few people knew she was having the baby and those who did thought she was married. As a result, she isolated herself from the young single women by letting them believe she was married and pretending to have nothing in common with them. She added that she knew she brought a lot of problems on herself because she had a need to hide her pregnancy and must now cover up what she has been through. She said she's not a liar by nature, but now finds herself telling lie after lie to keep people from finding out the truth.

Jane said she felt the same way. In fact, her parents went to the trouble of renting a post office box in the town where the camp was supposed to have been. They drove out there once a week to pick up her mail and drop off her responses so that no one would suspect anything. She also talked about how isolated she felt at the maternity home. Whenever she had a chance to go anyplace, she inevitably spotted a friend who she would have to avoid; as a result she spent most of her time inside. Betty said she also had to avoid people a lot. Once she stopped working she stayed in most of the time watching TV and having a miserable summer. She was so lonely and bored by the time the baby was born, she didn't know what to do with herself. After the baby was born, she decided to leave her old job and seek new employment rather than go on living a lie.

Both the process and the content of the early sessions were important to the development of the group. As the women became more aware of the similarities of their experiences, they became more comfortable talking about their feelings. They used the group to ventilate their feelings, consistently seeing themselves as victims. They were well defended, denying any responsibility for the difficulties they experienced while expressing anger and resentment towards those who had hurt them.

Most of the women in both groups had made some effort to hide their pregnancy from their families and friends for as long as possible in order to avoid the negative reactions they anticipated. Those who lived away from home and chose not to tell their families experienced a great deal of loneliness and isolation. They cut themselves off from whatever support their family might have provided. Those who remained at home eventually confided in their immediate family but concealed their pregnancy from their extended family and friends. One woman who remained in her community never left the house during the later stages of her pregnancy and was forced to retreat to her bedroom whenever guests came to visit.

The women who made no attempt to hide their pregnancy experienced other difficulties. They complained of being deluged by people giving them unsolicited advice, offering insensitive opinions, and expressing negative attitudes about unwed pregnancy. Similarly, some women reported spending most of their pregnancy surrounded by people who tried to ignore the pregnancy. They avoided any reference to the women's situation and dreaded the thought that there might be any discussion of the pregnancy whatsoever.

Not surprisingly, the women's description of their parents' attitudes towards the pregnancy, and their influence on the women's decision to surrender, were filled with ambivalence. Those members of the group whose parents were not accepting and supportive of their pregnancy commented that they were glad that their parents did not get too involved with their pregnancy or with their baby, since this might have made it difficult to give up the baby. However, subsequent expressions of anger and hostility towards their parents, in addition to ambivalence and regrets about their decisions, raised some questions about how much these women were rationalizing what had happened.

Others initially described a very accepting attitude on the part of their parents, but later confided that their parents had said things that evoked a great deal of resentment. To illustrate, during a discussion on how each client's parents reacted when they learned that their daughter was pregnant, one group member said that while sitting alone, watching television, her mother observed her overeating and asked if she were pregnant. When she admitted that she was, she was surprised at how accepting and comforting her mother was, noting that mother had even taken her shopping for maternity clothes the next day. She added that she was able to live at home throughout her pregnancy and got along okay with her mother. After hearing other group members talk about some of the negative experiences they had with their parents, however, this woman's mood gradually began to change, and she confided to the group that, in fact, later in her pregnancy she had also had a very unsettling experience with her mother. She told the group that her mother had said that while the decision to keep or surrender the baby was entirely hers, having raised eleven kids of her own, she couldn't be involved in handling another baby. If she decided to keep the baby, she would have to move out of the house.

During the discussions of their experience with their families it became clear that the issue of dependency vs. autonomy was central to many of the problems these women were having. While much of their behavior pointed to efforts to gain independence and become self-reliant, there was also a very apparent need to be nurtured and cared for. Many of the women who had left home prior to their pregnancy moved back during this period and some of those who did not explained that they were not welcomed. Those who lived at home seemed to find the thought of moving out on their own with a newborn baby much too threatening.

Reactions to the Decision to Surrender

Some of the women who came to the group felt they had worked through their feelings about surrendering their baby and the resulting adoption during their pregnancy. However, the birth of their baby renewed their ambivalence about these decisions. Those who had decided to surrender had second thoughts, and those who up until that point were sure they wanted to keep their baby began to have doubts. Without exception all of the women felt that reexamining their decision was one of the most difficult experiences of their lives. Often the difficulty seemed to be compounded by a variety of situations that occurred in the hospital, including efforts by some families and on occasion hospital staff, who tried to encourage or discourage them from seeing the baby during their stay. Overall, however, the group was united in its feeling that leaving the hospital without their babies was the most trying experience they had ever gone through.

A significant concern for all of these women was their perception of how people reacted to their decision. As workers explored these feelings, they began to see a great deal of anger over what the clients called the lack of concern and insensitivity of their parents, the alleged fathers, and peers. In many cases the alleged father initially denied paternity and abandoned the woman when she announced her pregnancy. Of those who acknowledged being the baby's father, few showed any interest or concern for the woman or the child. According to the women who attended the group, even those men who were willing to accept their responsibilities were not ready for marriage.

Reports of experiences with peers were equally negative. Many of the women felt that their peers were deliberately cruel. Abby had been questioning whether or not she had made the right decision and said she felt like a "martian" because girls in her town didn't give up their babies. She then told the group that while walking down the street she met a former classmate who was out for a walk with her baby. The two women had been pregnant about the same time but had made different decisions about whether to keep or surrender their children. Abby admired the other woman's baby and commented on how cute it was. Then, to show condemnation of women who surrender their babies for adoption, the woman looked Abby in the eye and said sarcastically, "Yes, I adopted her." The remark left Abby speechless, angry, and hurt. She then told the group she thought she was probably the only girl in her town who gave up her child.

The worst experiences, however, seem to be those that involved the client's family. There were reports of fathers who avoided any recognition or discussion of their daughter's pregnancy, and mothers who pressed their daughters to "stop crying and get back into the swing of things." Many of the women saw their decision to surrender their baby for adoption as a major failure, synonymous with incompetence, immaturity, and dependency.

> Debbie came to the group very ambivalent about having surrendered her baby for adoption. She told the group that her parents were very hurt and disappointed in her when they found out she was pregnant. In addition, because she had younger brothers and sisters, her parents did not allow her to stay at home during the pregnancy. They didn't want to see the baby in the hospital nor did they think Debbie should see her. Although her parents' reactions made her feel "really horrible," Debbie told the group that she was glad they didn't get

> too involved with her pregnancy nor with the baby, because it might have made it harder to give the baby up.
>
> As the group progressed, Debbie was able to express her feelings more openly. She confided that she really questioned whether or not she made the right decision. She wondered whether she might have been able to "make it with her baby." She spoke at length about her older sister who had an unwed pregnancy two years earlier. Significantly, Debbie's parents allowed her sister to stay at home during her pregnancy and have allowed her to live at home with her baby for the past two years. Debbie felt she had really been of help to her sister during the pregnancy. She expected her sister to do the same for her, but she didn't. Her sister wouldn't even talk to her about the pregnancy which made her feel hurt and rejected. Furthermore, seeing that her sister, who recently married, was doing so well caused Debbie to have some strong regrets about her decision to surrender. Unlike her sister, she never received the support or nurturance she longed for nor had she gained the recognition and independence she equated with becoming a parent.

Many of the women complained about the problems they had with their families. They were hurt and angry, but unable to acknowledge any responsibility for this. They were well defended and resisted efforts by the workers to explore and clarify the issues. As a result the workers maintained a supportive posture, acknowledging the sacrifices and hardships that the women had endured, while urging them to address their concerns more directly. Although most of the early interaction in the group was between the workers and individual clients, the group members gradually became more sensitive to each other's needs and better able to offer support and reassurance themselves. As the group progressed the members assumed more and more of the roles and responsibilities initially assumed by the workers. Not surprisingly, the women had a strong impact on each other. For some of them the support and encouragement they received from the group was incentive enough to enable them to confront family members and work through some of their problems.

> Nancy, for example, was repeatedly upset when her mother and a neighbor had long discussions about the neighbor's new baby. To Nancy, this seemed like a very insensitive and cruel

thing to do in her presence, since they never mentioned her baby or the experiences she had been through.

After several sessions had passed, Nancy told the group that as a result of the support she had received from them, she was able to talk to her mother about her feelings. Much to her surprise, she found her mother to be more sensitive and understanding than she had anticipated. More importantly, however, she was now able to join in the conversations with her family and friends and talk about her pregnancy and her child. She had begun to deal eith her own fears and insecurities and to recognize that her own problems were contributing to the difficulties she was experiencing.

The Middle Sessions

During the middle sessions the focus of the group began to shift. Gradually the group became more cohesive, and the members developed a more trusting relationship with each other and with the workers. At the same time, their concerns about problems with significant others diminished. They became more receptive to exploring their feelings and were able to examine their problems more objectively.

The change in focus began with the women raising questions about the welfare of their children, wondering how they were doing and whether or not surrendering them for adoption was the right decision. Exploring these concerns allowed the women to examine their feelings about adoption and adoptive parents and ultimately freed them to deal with their loss more directly.

In an effort to help the women work through some of these issues, the workers asked the group whether or not they might like to have an adoptive couple come to one of the sessions. Whether or not the couple ever came was not all that important, but discussing the possibility helped facilitate the group's taking a closer look at the issues and their feelings about them.

Self-Image

Discussions of adoption and concerns about having an adoptive couple attend a meeting helped one of the groups deal with issues of self-image. When the workers mentioned the option of having an adoptive couple come to the group, the women were hesitant. They were threatened by the possibility and suggested that "it might not be such a good idea." One woman wondered aloud what the group would say to an adoptive couple. Another said she'd be amazed if there was a couple who would be willing to come. As the discussion progressed, the real issue finally came to light: "What are they going to think of us, we all had babies and none of us are married." Similarly another woman said she also wondered, "What adoptive couples think of us, and if they don't think too highly of us, would their feelings be conveyed to the adopted child?" The group was finally able to express its concern about what other people think of unmarried mothers. They questioned their maturity, competency, and sexuality and they felt that they had lost the trust and respect of family and friends. Although they wanted to be seen as capable, responsible individuals, the experience of becoming pregnant and surrendering their baby created negative feelings about their sexuality and their ability to negotiate successfully adult relationships and fulfill adult responsibilities.

Grief and Loss

Prior to coming to the group many of the women had to one degree or another been unable to deal with their loss. Some felt guilty about giving up their baby but projected the guilt and blamed others—family, alleged fathers, caseworkers, or even "the agency—for making them give up their baby" or " not supporting them in their desire to keep the child." Others clung to the hope that adoption was not final and some day they'd be reunited with their "child." Some said they wanted to talk about what they had been through but no one cared enough to give them the opportunity. They found their families and friends to be insensitive and complained about not being given time to grieve with everyone encouraging them not to sit around and feel bad about what had happened.

Exploring the adoption issues proved to be a crucial aspect of helping the women deal more directly with their losses. When they began discussing the adoption issues, their first thoughts were of the child initiating an identity search resulting in their being reunited. A careful look at their fantasies revealed the picture of a young woman being reunited with an infant or child. Eventually, however, they began to feel that the chances of such a reunion occurring were very remote and that if it happened at all they would probably be middle-aged and their child would be an adolescent or young adult by the time such a reunion could occur. As part of the grief process they began to question their decision, expressed remorse about having given up their baby, and expressed a need to "suffer." Those who were not suffering expressed an overwhelming sense of guilt at not experiencing any pain.

> Another group's initial reaction to the workers' suggestion that they consider meeting with an adoptive couple was quite different.
>
> To their surprise the women were very receptive. The workers asked what the group would want to discuss with the couple, and they responded, "How do they tell a child he's adopted?" "When do they tell the child?" "Do the adoptive parents know that they didn't just give their child away?" They wanted them to know that they loved their children.
>
> Debbie wondered what an adoptive couple would do if their adopted child wanted to find its natural mother. This became the topic of conversation. Connie said she thinks the couple should let the child seek its (birth) mother. Violet said she agreed, she knows her child would never think of her as his parent, she knew he'd always think of the adoptive couple as his parents. She only hoped to be a friend to the child. The workers questioned whether they all had fantasies of their child returning. The group responded that they all did. The workers then asked how they thought this might happen. Connie pictured her son coming to her home, ringing her doorbell, and saying, "Hi, I'm your son." The workers asked how she would feel and she said she'd probably feel kind of funny, she's not really sure. Tina imagined the same thing. Violet said she'd like to get to know her son and be a friend to him. Debbie thought she'd have an immediate relationship between herself and her child. One of the workers commented that it seemed as if Debbie was picturing a small child coming back. Debbie said she was thinking of a child, adding that it was hard for her to think of her child grown up. The other worker commented that it seemed as if they're thinking of themselves as being the age they are now. Connie and Tina nodded their heads indicating they agreed. The workers then suggested that any reunion that might take place probably wouldn't happen for at least 18 years. Violet said that it was hard to accept it (the loss of her child) as absolutely final. Even a slim thread of

hope seemed better than nothing. She knows it may never happen, but she still hopes to be reunited. Connie said she didn't think she could have surrendered without some possibility of seeing her child someday. Tina and Debbie agreed with Connie's statement. Debbie said she can also see things from the adoptive parents point of view. If she adopted a child, she doesn't think she would want the child to look for his/her mother. Connie asked why, she said she knew she wouldn't change the relationship the child has with the adoptive parents, they've given the child life and security. Violet agreed. She said she can finally refer to the adoptive couple as "Kevin's parents," but it took her a long time to admit to herself that they would really be his parents, and not her. She would like to be his friend if he ever found her. Debbie feels that she still cannot accept that idea. She can't accept Kathy's adoptive family as her real parents, she still thinks of herself as the child's mother. She said now she really feels that she made the wrong decision. Then, beginning to cry, she added that she could have been a mother to her daughter.

Violet said she went through this too. She placed her child a year ago, then met a woman at work who was divorced when her child was a few months old. The woman raised the daughter herself. The girl is now 13 years old, into drugs, won't listen to her mother, and is seeing a psychiatrist. The mother really tried but things didn't work out. Violet said this could have happened to her, she knew she couldn't give her child the life she wanted him to have. She added that you can't do it without a husband and she's glad she didn't try. Debbie wished she could feel this way, but keeps thinking she could have done it. She now feels "depressed." Violet said she felt that way for a long time, but now she accepts her decision better, she feels that it was the right thing.

The group talked about how much they envied the fact that Violet "had it so together." The workers pointed out that each member was at a different stage of working through their loss, adding that Karen had experienced the same feelings that they were having, but she has had a year to work them out.

Connie said that she thought it would all be over when she signed the papers. Debbie said that she felt as if she's just beginning to have feelings about the placement. When she signed the papers, it didn't bother her that much. Connie agreed,

> noting that she was afraid to come to the group because she was fearful of thinking about adoption again. She felt that she had the situation under control, and new she has had to think about it again.

Both groups seemed to have similar experiences when they actually met with the adoptive couple. Although many of the women experienced a great deal of anxiety prior to the actual meeting, they became committed to taking advantage of the opportunity. During the meeting the group focused on a variety of issues:

1. What are adoptive couples like?
2. What are their motives for adopting?
3. What are their perceptions of birth mothers?
4. What would an adoptive couple tell their child about his/her birth mother?
5. What does this couple think of an adoption identity search?
6. What would the adoptive mother have done if she had had an unwed pregnancy?

The couple told the group that they had adopted because they were unable to have children of their own. They felt that they had a lot of love to share with a child and had found their life to be more fulfilled now that they had adopted their child. Much to the group's satisfaction, the couple indicated that they held the birth mother in high regard. They acknowledged how difficult it must be to surrender a child for adoption, feeling that a mother would have to love her child very much to make such an unselfish sacrifice. These sentiments also reflected what they thought they would tell their child when he/she began to ask about his/her birth mother.

Not all of the couples' comments were as well received. Even though they said that they would be perfectly comfortable with their child initiating an adopting identity search at an appropriate time, the group members later confided that they were not convinced that the adoptive couple would be so open-minded when they actually faced this situation.

The most threatening aspect of the group, however, was the adoptive mother's response to questions about what she would have done if she had experienced an unwed pregnancy. The woman said that she doubted that she would have been able to give up her baby. She then qualified her statements by saying that her own infertility definitely influenced her feelings and that she doubted that she could really give an objective response.

The remaining sessions were used to work through termination, but at the same time, the women tried to come to terms with their decision to surrender their babies. Some of them felt that they had gained a new understanding of themselves and what they had been through. Others indicated that they were more comfortable with themselves and could deal more effectively with the pregnancy, the surrender, and the reactions they encountered. A few felt that they were finally able to accept the loss of their children. They were now able to deal with their sadness and allow themselves to cry. All but one woman felt that just having someone to talk to about the experiences they had been through made the group worthwhile. One woman said that the group had been extremely painful for her. She said she dreaded coming to the group each week. When she was asked why she continued to come, she said that she was "looking for magic." Ironically, this same woman had told the group that signing the surrender papers didn't really bother her that much. In fact, it wasn't until halfway through the group that she actually began feeling badly about having placed her baby for adoption. Is it too much to suggest that those who find the group experience so difficult may be the ones who need it the most?

Unfortunately, there are no magical solutions to the problems faced by these clients, nor is the post-surrender group offered as a panacea. It is merely a modest attempt to provide an additional treatment option to a hard-to-reach client population. The need for extended services to women who surrender is indeed more urgent now than ever!

REFERENCES

Burgess, L. C. *The Art of Adoption.* Washington, D.C.: Acropolis Books, 1976.

Cheetham, J. *Unwanted Pregnancy and Counseling.* Boston: Routledge and Kegan Paul, 1977.

Garland, J. A., Jones, H. E., & Kolodny, R. L. A Model for Stages of Development in Social Work Groups. In S. Bernstein (Ed.), *Explorations in Group Work.* Boston: Charles River Books, 1976.

Grow, L. J. Today's Unmarried Mothers: The Choices Have Changed. *Child Welfare,* 1979, *6,* 363-371.

Nettleton, C. A. *A Search to Know How It Goes with You: A Follow-Up Study of Unmarried Mothers Who Have Made the Decision Regarding the Child.* Minnesota: Lutheran Social Services of Minnesota, 1972.

Roulet, N. Group Psychotherapy with Unmarried Mothers. In *The Double Jeopardy, The Triple Crisis, Illegitimacy Today*. New York: National Council on Illegitimacy, 1969.

Yalom, I. D. *The Theory and Practice of Group Psychotherapy*. New York: Basic Books, Inc., 1975.

Formulating Permanent Planning Strategies: Use of Group Decision Making by Key Professionals

Janet Lahti
Mary Troychak

ABSTRACT. The use of group processes in a series of residency institutes to formulate strategies to facilitate permanent planning is described. Key policymakers met to review data, list problems, and formulate plans. A total of 10 states participated, each sending between three and seven team members to a three-day session. Participants were chosen to represent a diversity of child welfare concerns. These residency institutes were conducted by staff of the national project to disseminate permanent planning methods. Results indicate a considerable interest in participating and a commitment to formulating plans which could be implemented.

The problem of children remaining for long periods in foster care has received increased attention during the past decade by those concerned with child welfare. Although it was designed as a way to provide a temporary home for children, foster care has all too frequently become an unplanned, long-term placement. An innovative approach addressing this issue, developed by the Permanent Planning Project at Portland State University's Regional Research Institute, involved a series of residency institutes which brought together key policymakers to plan necessary reforms. The focus was on the use of group processes for decision making. This paper will describe the organization and content of these institutes.

The problem of children remaining too long in foster care has been recognized for three decades. Since the late 1960s a number of projects have been conducted with the common goal of providing permanent homes for children in foster care, preferably by return-

Janet Lahti, PhD, is the Project Director for the Permanent Planning Project at the Regional Research Institute for Human Sciences, Portland State University. Mary Troychak, BA, is Research Assistant at the Institute.

ing them to their parents, and if this was not possible, seeking an adoptive placement (Emlen, 1976; Jones, 1977; Sherman, Neuman, and Shyne, 1973; Stein, 1978).

One of these projects initiated by Vic Pike (1976) culminated in the establishment of a national project to disseminate methods of securing permanent homes for children in agency care. Called the Permanent Planning Project, its focus was on providing technical assistance to states in their efforts to solve child welfare problems (Downs, 1981).

Based on the recognition that barriers to permanent planning and methods of overcoming them can appear from a number of sources, and with a desire to assist states in planning strategies of dealing with their problems, a series of institutes (hereafter called residency institutes) was held from November to May 1979-80, for key policymakers in child welfare from 10 states. The need for such a program was identified by Permanent Planning Dissemination Project field consultants working with individual states in an effort to institute needed child welfare reforms. They realized that in order to make certain changes necessary to improve child welfare practice input from professionals outside the social service agency would be useful. Selected professionals left their busy schedules to spend three days together in Portland, Oregon in an effort to formulate plans for needed change. What follows is a description of the residency institutes, with a focus on group process in the development of state plans to implement permanency planning for children.

Intense sessions were held for small, select groups. Group size was restricted in the belief that small group discussion would be more effective and efficient. Participants were chosen on the basis of demonstrated concern with the problem and ability to have an impact on solutions. Participants came from a number of disciplines, and thereby contributed diverse views of problems and abilities to formulate and expedite solutions. Developing a cohesive group had high priority and a number of activities were carried out with this goal in mind. The group activity was highly structured with the goal of reviewing data to identify problems, formulating solutions, and specifying plans for their implementation.

Organization

A group discussion method of decision making was chosen as a format for the sessions. One reason for this choice was the belief that a group of professionals, each of whom had expertise in a different facet of child welfare, would be more likely to formulate practical, workable solutions to child welfare problems than any individual working alone. Another reason for selecting a group discussion format was that members, each of whom came from a different discipline, would be likely to have an impact on a particular type of problem. For example, because of his experience with the courts, an attorney could initiate needed changes in court procedures. In this manner, a variety of problems could be addressed which might not be addressed by an individual. Group discussion was chosen for a third reason. It was a way to develop networks of key child welfare professionals who would know each other well enough to work together during the sessions as well as later. Open communication channels could be developed for carrying out the plans made at the residency institutes and perhaps to deal with new problems as they arose later (Schon, 1977).

Finally, if each group member gained a knowledge and understanding of problems, values, and behaviors of other members' professions this information could help unify diverse professions in working on common problems. If some transfer of technology could take place between attorneys and social workers, for example, each profession might benefit from being able to accomplish their goals more efficiently and effectively (Allen, 1977).

Selection of Participants

States were chosen to participate because there appeared to be a top level commitment to addressing the problem of protracted foster care. Participants from selected states were chosen because it seemed that they could make plans which they had the power to implement. While judgments of commitment and power are risky, the experience of the Permanent Planning Dissemination Project staff in working with a large number of states served as a basis on which to make these assessments and selections. This project and the residency institutes project were conducted by the Regional Research Institute at Portland State University, and the two were closely associated.

The selection process took place in the following way. An invitation to participate was sent to the commissioner of each state's social services agency. An acceptance of the invitation indicated at least some interest in taking action on child welfare problems. Throughout planning and conducting the institutes a practical approach was taken to assure that plans were not only made but acted upon. Of the 23 states making application, 10 were chosen to assemble a team of from three to seven participants. Team size was not allowed to exceed 12 in the belief that limiting the size would increase the extent and quality of the communication (Hare, 1952). Once a state was chosen, the commissioner responsible for that state's social service agency designated a person, usually the head of that state's foster care program, to put together the state team. Teams from two states attended each one of the five sessions. Team selection was done in cooperation with permanent planning staff and the director of the residency institutes project. A list was made of persons who had demonstrated an interest in and commitment to working on child welfare problems. From this list invitations were issued to those seen as best able to formulate and carry out plans for change. Teams selected were represented by administrators in a state social service agency, legislators, school of social work faculty who teach child welfare, representatives from the legal profession such as law professors, attorneys general, private practitioners, or judges active in juvenile law, and leaders in child advocacy groups such as foster parent associations or citizen task forces on the rights of children.

Structure

Because it seemed likely that high level professionals would only be able to spend a limited time away from their state, a three-day residency institute was held. Activity was intense during this period, sessions lasted all day, individual conferences were fit into any spare time, and informal gatherings occupied the evenings.

In the belief that issues could be more thoroughly and openly explored in a relaxed and cordial environment, an effort was made from the beginning to set this tone. On the evening of the participants' arrival an informal gathering was held in the home of one of the permanent planning staff for state teams and for staff participating in the institutes.

Participants were reminded that taking a role as a peer in a problem-solving group might mean a role change for some of them. For some, it meant stepping out of an administrative role in a familiar discipline and becoming a group member with persons from another range of experiences; agency administrators must communicate with juvenile court judges and legislators must communicate with child advocacy group leaders.

Except for the information sessions described below and a short session at the end of the residency institutes during which teams reported their plans and strategies to each other, the teams met separately. Three staff members from the Permanent Planning Project met with each team; an attorney served as a resource person on legal issues; the field consultant having primary responsibility for permanent planning activities in that state participated as a team member; and another field consultant acted as a facilitator whose task it was to be certain all issues were explored and plans and strategies developed. One of the state team members recorded the group activities and prepared a report.

Content

Two kinds of activities took place. One was a capsule presentation of the nature of the child welfare problem to be addressed, efforts made to deal with the problem, and the results of these efforts. The purpose of this presentation was to develop basic understanding of the problem among residency institute participants and to give them a broad perspective as they identified problems and sought solutions. A second kind of activity involved group discussion by team members and was designed to survey the nature of the foster care problem in their states, work out solutions, and make plans for implementing the desired change. This decision-making process will be described in what follows.

A three-step process was undertaken to help states conclude at the end of the three days with the desired plans and strategies. First, the teams reviewed data available from their own state. To accomplish this, a questionnaire was sent to all participants prior to the residency institutes requesting the following information: whether the social service agencies are administered, supervised, and funded by the state or county; the number, average age, and average length of time in care for foster children in the state; the annual expenditure in the state for foster care services; the options for exiting from foster care; the number of children in the state returned to their biological parents from foster care last year; the services to children available in the state; the criteria for labelling a child "hard to place"; the number of adoption placements presently receiving subsidy; and whether or not the state has a case review system. Participants reviewed these data together at the beginning of the team sessions. The questionnaires had the effect not only of giving participants a basis for decision making but also had the somewhat unexpected effect of making them aware of any knowledge that was now available which would have been useful to decision making. The plans of a number of states included obtaining these data. For some states the absence of such data as the number, age, and average stay in foster care pointed to the need for the development of such elements in an information system.

From problems identified by reviewing questionnaire data and from the knowledge of residency institute participants about their state, barriers to permanent planning were identified and systematically recorded. A selection of those barriers to receive attention was then made as a second step. The criteria used to select problems for attention by the team were that the problem was an important impediment to permanent planning and that a solution seemed possible. As an example of this process, one state determined that a change in its termination of parental rights statute would be desirable. After considering the chances of succeeding in instituting such a change in view of the fact that a revision to the law (considered by the team to be unacceptable) had been made at the last legislative session, the team decided to shelve efforts to make this change. Instead, they chose to seek other ways of overcoming the identified barriers and plans were made to seek legislative change at a later time.

Once problems to receive attention were chosen, specific solutions were planned by the team. Because an effort would be made to implement the desired changes, a realistic plan was of prime importance. Team members considered the possible alternative solutions to the problem and chose the one which seemed most desirable and had good prospects for implementation. After a plan for overcoming barriers was formulated, the third step was to develop strategies to implement these plans. This meant formulating a step-by-step action plan as well as designating who would be responsible for implementation at each step. Finally, a report of these plans and strategies was presented to residency institute participants and staff.

In summary, the focus of the residency institutes was a practical one. In the beginning, data were collected to identify the nature of the problem. Teams were chosen for their expertise in addressing such problems and for their ability to have an impact on solutions. To be sure, one important outcome was the realization that, in some instances, data useful to decision making did not exist and this in itself suggested changes. Data were discussed and from this discussion barriers to permanent planning were identified. Specific workable solutions were planned. Finally, tasks were allocated to team members and time lines developed for implementing the plan.

Results

The results of an endeavor such as this one can best be assessed by determining the extent to which the goals were achieved. The overall goal of permanent planning efforts is to assure that each child receiving agency services is receiving those services as a part of an overall time-limited plan, designed to provide him with a permanent home. Of course, it would be naive to expect a single three-day effort to achieve this goal. There were, however, some reasonable objectives related to this goal which perhaps could be met. One was to promote and consolidate high level and diversified support within the states for permanency planning. Another was for each team to develop a plan to solve their child welfare problems with strategies for its implementation. Of course, whether or not that plan got carried out was of interest. However, any success, or failure, in achieving objectives could not be solely attributed to the residency institutes. The influence of such factors as other individuals and groups in a state, the political climate, changes in agency funding, and changes in agency administration can make a difference in how plans are carried out. With these limitations in mind, the results of the residency institutes were evaluated in several ways.

A number of methods were used to assess whether the objective of promoting high level and diversified support was met. The first indicator was the extent to which a team of high level persons could be assembled. Participants included 16 state agency administrators; nine legislators with a demonstrated interest in child welfare issues; seven school of social work faculty; nine representatives from the legal profession; six leaders in child advocacy groups; and one regional representative from the U.S. Health and Human Services Children's Bureau.

Given the willingness of such participants to attend the residency institutes, their feelings about the sessions could be another indicator of the likelihood that they supported permanency planning. Team ratings seemed to indicate satisfaction with the residency institutes. Participants were asked to rate each separate activity on a scale from one (''not useful'') to four (''very useful''). The median overall response was 3.5. Ratings of the group planning and strategy sessions ranged from 3.0 to 3.86.

Also related to promoting high-level, diversified support for permanent planning was the objective of developing networks among individuals who could institute foster care reform in their states. The residency institutes environment was one in which professionals concerned with child welfare could air their views, learn of the trials and accomplishments of their colleagues, become acquainted with the nationwide effort, and develop a state plan. Coming together in this setting permitted the participants to establish a network of contacts outside their respective professions which they could, perhaps, pursue later. Lawyers became acquainted with agency administrators, judges were confronted with the problems and perspectives of child advocates, social work faculty were exposed to the daily issues confronting social work practitioners. In some instances, the teams continued to function as a network or as a more formally structured task force to implement the state plan, but the exact manner and extent of network functioning following the residency institutes is not known.

The second objective, to develop a plan for foster care reform and a strategy for its implementation, can be assessed more directly. The first step was identifying the barriers to permanent planning within the state. Table 1 summarizes the defined barriers. It can be noted that considerable similarity existed among states regarding perceived barriers to permanent planning. The need for caseworker training, for legal representation, and for a useful management information system were seen as problems by the largest number of states.

No such similarity existed in the plans developed by the states for overcoming the barriers. Plans for dealing with an inadequate termination of parental rights statute, for example, varied from planning a complete revision of the statute to developing political strategy for getting a previously revised version passed by the legislature.

The strategies developed for beginning the effort to carry out the plan were somewhat similar and seem to indicate a commitment to implementation as well as certain political skills. To begin implementation, five states planned to arrange a conference with the commissioner of the social service agency who had indicated an interest in addressing foster care problems by arranging for team participation in the residency institutes. This meeting was to report team discussions and recommendations formulated during the residency institutes. This action was prompted by the belief that

TABLE 1

Permanent Planning Barriers

Defined by State Teams*

Barrier	Number of States
Caseworkers need training	8
Agency lacks legal representation	7
Lack of a useful management information system	6
Inadequate termination of parental rights statute	5
Lack of funds for child welfare services	4
Case review method is undeveloped	4
Agency has insufficient commitment to permanent planning	3
State does not have a written policy on permanent planning	3
State policies do not promote permanent planning goals	3
Agency staff unwilling to terminate parental rights	3
Agency staff unwilling to permit foster parent adoption	3
Adoption subsidy is inadequate or not used	3
No funding for families to adopt hard to place children	3

*Barriers listed are those identified by at least three states.

some plans could be implemented, or at least the beginnings of implementation achieved, if the commissioner would make a commitment in principle to the plan. Five states planned to request that the team be the nucleus of a task force appointed to implement the plan.

One barrier, the lack of agency commitment to permanent planning, could be addressed by a statement of support by the commissioner. While solutions required more than a verbal commitment, this was considered to be the beginning. Beyond the point of meetings with the commissioner, the specific plans of the states varied widely. It was evident from examining them that these were practical plans, specific to the state situations.

The residency institutes were also evaluated in terms of the extent to which plans were carried out. Although all kinds of things not associated with the quality of the plan itself or the dedication of team members can obstruct or facilitate implementation, a general judgment is possible.

A survey was conducted two months after the residency institutes for the purpose of measuring progress toward goals. Results indicate that every state had made progress on at least half of their goals and nine of the 10 participating states had achieved one or more goals. No single type of goal appears more difficult to achieve than another. Getting legislation passed to change a state's termination of parental rights statute seems to have been no more easy or difficult than instituting a tracking system for foster care cases.

Conclusions

The Residency Institutes demonstrated that it is possible to use group processes with key policymakers to formulate workable plans for child welfare reform. The components of the method which seem most relevant are: the use of interdisciplinary groups, selecting as participants key professionals in positions to influence policy, maintaining a small group size, developing a cohesive group, and the use of a structured decision-making format.

The scope of the discussion was broadened by the presence of interdisciplinary teams. Each person brought a special knowledge and expertise which added dimension to the problem-solving process. By considering such diverse viewpoints, workable solutions were more likely to follow. When it came to implementing the plan, having support from a number of sources gave the plan creditability and increased its chances of being implemented.

By selecting as participants those in positions to understand and influence policy, the chances of having an impact increased. These were people who were experienced in policy formulation and could assess the advisability of attempting a policy change. They were willing and able to focus their divergent viewpoints to develop a plan that seemed workable.

Keeping the size of the group small contributed to efficiency and effectiveness. Time was short and the task of reviewing a state child welfare system and designing reforms was a difficult one. In a small group, participants could get acquainted more quickly and know each other better.

An effort was made to develop a group atmosphere in which participants had a commitment to cooperating with each other in accomplishing the task. Such group cohesion seemed important in facilitating the formulation of a workable plan and for influencing the success of the implementation effort. This was accomplished in several ways. The fact that the work of each state team was taken seriously seemed to help develop a sense of group purpose and strength. The effort was not merely an exercise. It was a serious attempt to address important child welfare problems. Focusing on the development of a plan to which each team member was committed seemed to add to group solidarity. The informal atmosophere maintained throughout the residency institutes seemed to develop group cohesion and provide an environment where open discussion could take place. For some, this meant a willingness to abandon temporarily the rather formal role taken in their daily profession.

The structured decision-making framework was important to the residency institutes. It involved asking participants to collect data ahead of time, discuss the data, identify problems indicated by the data, and develop solutions and strategies for implementing them. It was a practical approach, taken seriously by both staff and participants. Each state team left with a plan for needed child welfare reform as well as a timetable of strategies for its implementation.

REFERENCES

Allen, T. The role of person to person communication networks in the dissemination of industrial technology. Prepared for the Networking Conference sponsored by the School Capacity for Problem Solving Group, National Institute of Education: Washington, D.C., March 16-17, 1977.

Downs, S. *Foster Care Reform in the 70's: Final report of the permanency planning dissemination project.* Portland, Oregon: Regional Research Institute for Human Services, Portland State University, in press.

Emlen, A. *Barriers to planning for children in foster care.* Portland, Oregon: Regional Research Institute for Human Services, Portland State University, 1976.

Gordon, H. L. Long-time care. *Child Welfare,* January 1950, 3-8.

Gordon, H. L. *Casework services for children: Principles and practices.* Boston: Houghton Mifflin, 1956.

Gruber, A. *Children in foster care: Destitute, neglected, betrayed.* New York: Human Sciences Press, 1978.

Hare, P. A. A study of interaction and consensus in different sized groups. *American Sociological Review,* 1952, *17,* 261-267.

Jenkins, S. Duration of foster care: Some relevant antecedent variables. *Child Welfare,* 1967, *46,* 450-455.

Jones, M. L. Aggressive adoption: A program's effect on a child welfare agency. *Child Welfare,* 1977, *56,* 401-407.

Lahti, J. *Adoption of children in foster care: A comparison of processes leading to adoption by foster parents and adoption by others.* (Doctoral Dissertation, Portland State University, 1979). *Dissertation Abstracts International,* 1980, *40,* 4748A. (University Microfilms No. 800-3083)

Lewis, M. E. Long time temporary placement. *Child Welfare,* 1951, *30,* 307.

Maas, H. Children in long-term foster care. *Child Welfare,* 1969, *48,* 321-333.

Maas, H. S. and Engler, R. *Children in need of parents.* New York: Columbia University Press, 1959.

Pike, V. A. Permanent planning for children in foster care: The Oregon project. *Children Today,* November-December 1976.

Schon, D. A. *Network-related intervention.* Boston, Massachusetts: Massachusetts Institute of Technology, Department of Urban Studies and Planning, August 1977.

Sherman, E. A., Newman, R., and Shyne, A. *Children adrift in foster care: A study of alternative approaches.* New York: Child Welfare League of America, 1973.

Stein, T. J., Gambrill, E. D., and Wiltse, K. T. *Children in foster homes: Achieving continuity of care.* New York: Praeger, 1978.

Weissman, I. Children in long-term foster care. *Child Welfare,* June 1950, 3-7.

Staff Planning Groups: Internal Advocates of Permanency Planning for Children in Foster Care

Philip Villone

ABSTRACT. An analysis of a staff planning group established to expedite "permanency planning"* by the integration of services offered by two divisions within a public child welfare agency.

Any organization, including a social agency, may be viewed as a mosaic of interacting groups or systems. With the exception of a few administrative journals, the social work literature has largely ignored the existence of staff planning groups, often referred to as committees. As Olmsted has pointed out, "the plans and decisions which guide large scale enterprises in this country are in good part made by committees and conferences."[1] This is particularly true in the social welfare field today and has special import for the larger bureaucratic agencies. Rapidly shifting priorities in the delivery of services, dictated by governmental mandates and funding considerations, have heightened the prominence of such groups.

While the role of "internal advocacy" has traditionally been viewed as "initiated in the lower reaches of the administrative hierarchy," mandate by upper level administration for staff planning groups can boost the effectiveness of the advocacy role of practitioners as well as their importance in agency decision making.[2] The use of a group taps those attributes that Patti and Resnick note to be valuable in effecting change: "cosmopolitan orientation," i.e., a

Philip Villone, CSW, ACSW, is Supervisor II at SSC Division of Adoption and Foster Care Services, New York, New York.

*Permanency planning, as used here, refers to the timely return of the child to his/her biological or extended family, or where this is not feasible, to an adoptive home. It is recognized that for some children placed in foster care, neither of these objectives is a viable option and permanent foster homes may be considered as the only plan offering any semblance of permanence.

commitment to professional values and norms together with affiliation with others who have the same commitment; "informal leadership," i.e., having linkages with several subgroups within the agency; "educational or experiential qualifications," i.e., performance of specialized tasks within the agency; and "specialized information or knowledge."[3]

This article will deal with the group in an internal advocacy role, as a subsystem of the broader agency system, and with the impact on the individuals who comprised the group as well as their interaction with the broader agency system.

The Task

In January 1980, the Office of Direct Child Care Services, an administrative unit of the New York City, Human Resources Administration, Special Services for Children Agency, set out to reorganize its foster care and adoption services in an effort to expedite permanency planning for children served by the Division of Foster Home Care and the Division of Adoption Services. The two divisions involved operated as distinct subunits of the Office of Direct Child Care Services with each delivering specific permanency services. The problem areas identified by Administration were:

1. Delays in discharge plan implementation for children who were to be returned to biological/extended family.
2. Delays in the adoption study process for children who were legally free for such planning after a decision that reunion with biological/extended family was not feasible.
3. An imbalance of different level line staff in the two divisions and an imbalance in workload in the four office locations encompassed by the two divisions.

The Director of the Office of Direct Child Care Services (ODCCS) made the decision to utilize a staff planning group as a first step in the formulation of a plan to integrate the foster care and adoption services.

The staff planning group would be expected to provide recommendations for changes within the broader system encompassed by the two divisions, with the final decision-making responsibility remaining with the ODCCS Director and his superiors. The group was instructed by the Director "to focus on changes in structure, process, and staffing patterns that will lead to the provision of unified services to the children in care." Also to be addressed were training needs and plans for stages of implementation for any recommended changes. The group was assigned a three-and-one-half week period in which to address the task, with no limitations upon the frequency or duration of meetings. The time period was extended, subsequently, to eight weeks.

Group Composition

The group membership was mandated to consist of a specific representative cross section of personnel from each of the two divisions. Patti refers to this as "selective involvement" and states that "in an organization of any size and complexity, the administrator must make judgements about which practitioners can meaningfully contribute to the resolution of which issues."[4] The concept of designation of participants to be involved in a planning group is not unlike quota systems or screening criteria used in other social work or psychotherapy groups to determine composition.

The actual participants were not selected by the Director, but rather, in most instances, were volunteers from the two divisions. The Division of Foster Home Care, with a staff totaling 239, was allotted nine participant slots in the group. The representative members included: a location Director, a level III Supervisor, a level II Supervisor, two level I Supervisors, two Caseworkers and two Clerical Supervisors. The Division of Adoption Services, with a staff totaling 48, was allotted seven participant slots in the group. Its representative members included: a location Director, a level III Supervisor, a level II Supervisor, two level I Supervisors, a Caseworker and a Clerical Supervisor. In addition, a consultant/observer from the Office of Staff Development and Training was invited to be present at the group meetings to identify training needs and resources in relation to any envisioned changes.

The date, time and location of the first planning group meeting were established by the ODCCS Director. The location designated for the meetings was the conference room of the Division of Adoption Services.

The First Meeting

The planning group members arrived within twenty minutes after the starting time for the first scheduled meeting. A series of tables had been arranged as an open rectangle with an empty space in its center. It was observed that members tended to seat themselves next to other people from their office locations, confirming the existence of pregroup alliances. The two Directors sat at opposite ends of the rectangle from one another. This seating pattern remained essentially the same for the duration of the group. Since no leader had been designated, several minutes elapsed during which people conversed informally. At some point, one of the office Directors indicated that the meeting should be convened. Other members quickly responded, making suggestions about how to proceed. The members verbalized a consensus that two chairpersons should be elected to lead the group. Nominations were made and a "show of hands" vote taken; a level II Supervisor and a Caseworker were selected as the chairpersons. Interestingly, both the leaders selected were from the Division of Foster Home Care and both were elected with support from members of both divisions.

The first step taken by the group leaders was to get those present to introduce themselves. Members were asked to give their names, their job titles, a short statement as to how they perceived the group and its charge from upper administration, and their feelings about the prospect of a major programmatic change. All of those present articulated some fear about the impact of any change on their job functioning, as well as skepticism about the reasons "Administration" had decided to involve them in the planning process. Many members expressed the suspicion that the group's involvement in the planning task was a "tour de force" in that an administrative plan may already have been developed. Paradoxically, everyone agreed that his or her reason for volunteering to participate in the group was predicated on the hope and prospect that the group's input would have an impact on the final services integration plan. General agreement was articulated that the two services, adoption and foster care, had to be changed to better serve the children for whom they were responsible and to expedite the flow of planning activity. A certain degree of mutuality was apparent by virtue of the fact that all members present had volunteered to take on the task to be addressed by the planning group and verbalized a common objective; what was not yet verbalized were the conceptual goals to achieve the stated objective. Alliances were already apparent in the seating arrangement, and it was known that broad philosophical differences were operating between the two divisions involved. Hartford refers to this clearly:

> Interest alliances frequently shift and change in the course of a session related to an issue under consideration or the activity of

a group. On the other hand they make for strong factional divisions in a group that play into all of the processes of deliberation and decision making.[5]

One of the group leaders reflected back to the group the common concerns and expectations they as individuals had verbalized. The introductions and recapitulation of shared concerns and objective seemed to dispel much of the tension. Some informal comments were exchanged between members across the table as well as between those seated next to one another. After a few minutes, the question was raised of where to begin. One of the leaders suggested looking at the present service work flow in relation to the individual office locations and between the two divisions, to identify problem areas. This step was supported by the members. A series of flow charts was drawn on a blackboard, indicating the entry of children into foster care and adoption, as well as the process of securing foster and adoptive homes. Discussion ensued about the perceived pros and cons of the existing work flow. The group also began to look at obstacles to service in their existing office structures. Philosophical differences emerged between members of the two divisions about how problem areas were to be prioritized and about how to eliminate obstacles to the work flow.

A heated exchange between a foster care Supervisor and an adoption Supervisor occurred when the work flow of children between the two divisions was discussed. Accusations and counteraccusations were made by the two members; terminology such as "you people" reflected some deep-seated adversary positions among members. One of the group leaders intervened, pointing out that personal invectives were not a solution to alleviating conflicting viewpoints and philosophical differences. Members from both divisions supported the group leader. They also encouraged the two group members involved in the verbal interchange to negotiate differences as they related to the group task, not on an individual personality level. This group norm had to be reaffirmed on many subsequent occasions by both the leaders and membership in ensuing meetings.

Before the end of the first meeting, the issues of subsequent meetings and duration of the group were discussed. While it was pointed out by the group leaders that the group had only been given three and one-half weeks to complete its task, the members were reluctant to meet more than once each week, indicating that their participation in the group took time away from their service responsibilities. The members also suggested that since the next meeting was scheduled for the morning, they would like to have an urn of coffee set up. A collection was taken with one group leader and a member from the Division of Adoption Services agreeing to make the necessary arrangements for the next meeting. Since the group had limited time to submit its recommendations, the group leaders suggested that it would be helpful if each office prepared data for the next meeting indicating their present structures, staffing patterns and workload (population of children served). The members agreed to this as well as to solicit recommendations from all levels of staff in their respective locations, about changes in the service structures.

Role of Group Leaders

After the first meeting, the two group leaders met to discuss the meeting and to define their functions at future group sessions. Both were concerned about the factional differences between the two divisions, which held potential for personal antagonisms between group members. The name-calling between two members, which had erupted during the first session, could have severely impaired the group's task functioning if it had gone unchecked. Both leaders agreed that emotionally charged conflicts around issues were to be both expected and necessary, but that supports had to be established to keep the group focused upon their task. The leaders decided to rotate as the "instrumental leader" of the group.[6] While one leader would take responsibility for the cognitive problem-solving task of the group, the other would attempt to provide the affective monitoring of the group and be prepared to intervene if emotional conflicts between members became too intense. They perceived these two roles as particularly critical during the initial phase of group development. They also decided to meet before and after subsequent group sessions to reassess their co-leadership.

The Second Meeting

The second group meeting began only a few minutes after its scheduled starting time. Members from each of the offices distributed the data requested at the previous meeting. It was apparent that a good deal of time and effort had been expended on this task. The coffee urn had been set up as the group had requested.

The instrumental leader for that meeting placed the structural charts for each of the offices on the blackboard. Operating concepts in relation to the flow charts presented at the previous meeting, were presented at the blackboard by a member from each of the offices. Discussion about the viability of the structures in relation to service needs was lively. There was agreement that while the structures presented were in many ways similar, some offered innovations which expedited the permanency planning process. Staffing factors were also discussed since both divisions had been reduced in size by a combination of attrition and a hiring freeze which had been in effect for several years.

When the group began to focus on the interface of permanency planning between the two divisions, pronounced philosophical differences again emerged between members. One major area of agreement was that children being adopted by their foster families would be better served if they remained with the foster care worker through the entire study. Discussion was particularly heated, however, around the issue of children referred to the Division of Adoption Services for adoption by other than their foster families. There was, however, no further use of invectives and the members appeared to respect the convictions, if not viewpoints, of each other.

Towards the end of the meeting, there was a fairly lengthy discussion about how the group would resolve areas where there was no consensus for recommendation to the ODCCS Director. It was eventually suggested that the group, which was composed of an unequal number of members from each of the two divisions, could present options as a way of reflecting areas of contention in the final plan. It was also recognized that the fewer these areas, the stronger the plan. The group also agreed to meet the following week for a full day since the allotted time was almost depleted.

The Third through Fifth Meetings

Over the next two weeks, three meetings were held, each for a full day. An assessment of the needs of the service system and changes of procedure were focused upon. A great deal of time was also spent trying to compile and reconcile child planning statistics. By the fourth meeting it became apparent that additional time was needed by the group to meaningfully address the task of evolving a comprehensive services integration plan. The group decided to prepare a report to the ODCCS Director, identifying the recommendations to date and requesting additional time for the planning group to complete its charge. The ODCCS Director, upon receipt of the report, agreed to extend the planning group for another month.

The Sixth Meeting

From the beginning of the sixth meeting of the group, all of the members were noticeably tense. Between the fifth and sixth meetings, the members had reported those changes recommended to the ODCCS Director to their location staff. The reactions of staff to many of the proposed changes was vociferously negative in some instances, and the group members' moods reflected those reactions of their colleagues. The reports to staff within the various offices had, prior to now, gotten little, if any, attention. One at a time, the members related to the group the accusations of their fellow staff members that they had "sold out." Pressure from several levels of staff within the respective offices were recounted. One member said, "My people see me as some sort of traitor. They think we're all crazy." The impact on the members from the Division of Adoption Services was intensified because the group met in their conference room. Several members shared their feelings of pressure from co-workers every time they left the meeting room. Going to the bathroom often meant being subjected to questions about what was going on in the group. Patti points out that "the practitioner who confronts a potential advocacy situation is inevitably faced with making an assessment of the personal risks involved."[7] The members of the planning group were experiencing the consequences of taking such risks. In the statements made by almost every group member, the conflict of alliances was evident. The broader agency system was, literally, where the group members lived. Patti notes that:

> Membership in the system refers not simply to the criterion of employment, but to whether the practitioner is perceived as being an integral part of the group life of the institution (and is) more crucially dependent upon an incumbent's understanding of the organization's normative structure, both formal and informal, its ideology and its vested interests.[8]

The group members tended to be very supportive of one another in the face of this type of pressure. It appeared at this point that the group had become cohesive and that the broad differences evident in the earlier meetings had been ameliorated. The group reaffirmed its conviction that changes in the service structure had to be aimed at providing better service to its client population, within the limits of the available resources. It was recognized that any plan for service integration would result in broader responsibilities for all levels of staff as well as an increased workload. The group identified a major obstacle to its task as the unavailability of statistics identifying the positions of children in the permanency planning phases. Such statistics were deemed necessary to finalize certain structural changes (i.e., number of service teams needed for each phase of permanency planning) as well as to assess the impact of such statistics on projected phases of implementation of the plan for integration of the two divisions. It was decided that the next few meetings would have to focus upon this area, and members agreed to have full day meetings twice each week until the group's task was complete. Four of the members, including the two Directors, then added that they would not be able to attend meetings during the next one to two weeks. With the agreement of those members, the group decided to continue to meet without them.

The Seventh through Ninth Meetings

The group, reduced by four members, appeared to operate more spontaneously and required less direction from the group leaders during the seventh through ninth meetings. Recommendations were made about the provision of adoption services to children legally free for adoption residing in foster homes, where the present foster parents did not wish to adopt. Three options were presented by members to expedite the planning for such children, each representing a different conceptual orientation and each having different ramifications for the workloads within an integrated program. There was a great deal of discussion about the new organizational structures that would be required by the merger of the two divisions. Enthusiasm was evident in the group, despite their continued lack of success in obtaining the needed statistics identifying their target population. Timeframes of permanency planning activity were analyzed and discussed. Other staff members, from the different offices involved, were invited to attend the eighth meeting to share their recommendations for the integration of services. The group worked diligently during the week and one-half encompassing the three meetings. The group leaders, in their postgroup discussions, attributed this in part to the smaller size of the group and the absence of the two location Directors. Patti, in discussing the limitations of internal advocacy, points out that

> although participatory management is necessary and desirable, it tends to be inherently limited as a vehicle for the exercise of practitioner influence and may serve to divert worker initiated change efforts.[9]

The Tenth Meeting

Only one member was absent from the tenth group meeting. Those members present during the previous three meetings recapitulated the areas covered by the group for the members who had been absent. This process used much of the group's time since rationales for decisions often had to be explained to those members who had not been present. Although this back-tracking took an entire morning, by the afternoon the group was ready to begin finalizing the integrated service structures for each of the offices. There was heated debate about the concept of shared cases and the idea of having more than one practitioner involved in the planning for a child. It was generally recognized that as two divisions with distinct services, this process had not worked. Some members contended that with the merging of the two divisions into one, this principle could work. Other members countered that only in rare circumstances should the planning for a child be done by more than one practitioner. There was a clear dichotomy on this issue between the members from the Division of Adoption Services and those from the Division of Foster Home Care, and the way this issue was resolved would have impact on the final office structures and workload of staff in the offices.

Invectives were again passed between the same two members who tangled during the second session. One of the leaders attempted to intervene but was ignored by the group members who had all begun to verbalize personal antagonisms towards each other. After several minutes, the group began to settle down, and one of the leaders successfully intervened to refocus the group on its task. One of the members involved in the initial altercation apologized to the other member involved and the others supported this gesture. The group leaders reminded those present of the early agreement to offer the ODCCS Director a report on their areas of dissension along with their recommendations. One member expressed a strong opinion that the group should not submit options in its integration proposal, since that would weaken the credibility of the planning group's recommendations. While the other members agreed with the intent of that idea, they expressed doubt that consensus could be achieved in all areas.

After further group discussion, three similar but distinct service models and organizational structures were proposed. There was agreement that all three models would be presented in the planning group's final report, together with the rationales for each. Group members advocating each of the three models were encouraged to develop the rationales and present them for incorporation in the services integration plan report which would be forwarded to the ODCCS Director. The group agreed to use the next sessions to look at staffing considerations and needs using the three options and service models proposed. What also remained to be discussed were the stages for implementation of the integration of services and the other recommendations involved in the logistics of the service integration (i.e., training, shifting of staff and telephones, etc.).

The Eleventh through Thirteenth Meetings

Although the decision had tentatively been made in the tenth meeting to submit all three service integration proposals to the ODCCS Director, members did use these subsequent meetings to attempt to gain support for their preferred models. Members were exposed to continued pressure within their office locations to coerce the group to accept a preferred model. There was general discontent among staff in all of the offices of the two divisions about all three of the suggested models, since all contained concessions to accommodate the philosophical and conceptual differences between the two divisions. Work on the stages of implementation and the other recommendations proceeded smoothly and rapidly during these two meetings. One area of continued friction was about the numbers of children who would be planned for by the different offices under the integration plan. It was recognized that the foster care division would suffer the greatest increase in workload initially, in order to reduce the service backlog which would be inevitable when the two divisions merged. This was by no means an easy pill for the foster care staff or for the members of the planning group from that division to swallow.

The Fourteenth Meeting

The final scheduled planning group meeting was marked by last-minute efforts to arrive at a consensus about one service model. These efforts proved fruitless, and all three models with their rationales would be incorporated into the report to the ODCCS Director. A good deal of the group's time was spent editing the rationales for each of the models and reviewing the other recommendations. The group leaders offered to take responsibility for writing the report. Because there was no remaining time, the group members agreed but indicated that they wished to review the report before its submission to Administration. Although this was only five days before the expiration of the group's mandate, the leaders agreed to present the entire report to the group the day before it would be given to the Director.

The Final Meeting

During this final, somewhat anticlimactic meeting the members were subdued while reviewing the finished products of their labors. The members expressed their knowledge that many of the recommendations were unpopular, but there was general consensus that they had given the task their "best shot." A few corrections were made on the final report, and it was quickly approved for submission. The group members acknowledged their appreciation of the efforts of the two group leaders to finalize the report, and the meeting ended. Group members lingered in the meeting room, and a few were heard commenting about how strange it would be to not meet any longer. While everyone verbalized relief over completing the task, the final meeting was marked by a mood of sadness. Even though the group had not been able to arrive at a total consensus, the recommendations made indicated a convergence of opposing thoughts and values.

Conclusion

While staff planning groups hold promise for internal advocacy, they do have limitations as demonstrated by the described group experience. Within every system there is resistance to change. The resistance of staff in the broader agency system to any change in the service system had a profound impact on the members of the planning group. That powerful, pervasive resistance limited the ability of the group to negotiate and resolve all of the issues presented to it before submitting its report to upper Administration. The resistances and conflicts evidenced within the planning group foreshadowed what would occur during the actual services integration process.

Although the task-oriented group described here might not be considered as falling within Papell and Rothman's "mainstream model" of social work groups, it did possess many of the attributes of that model as well as of the "structured group" approach.[9] The group evidenced the stages of development, dynamics, and most of the other elements common to social work groups more often discussed in the literature.

NOTES AND REFERENCES

1. Michael S. Olmsted. *The Small Group.* New York: Random House, 1959, p. 86.
2. R. J. Patti. Limitations and Prospects of Internal Advocacy. *Social Casework, 55* (November 1974), p. 537.
3. Rino J. Patti and Herman Resnick. Changing the Agency from Within. *Social Work, 17* (July 1972), p. 52.
4. R. J. Patti, *op. cit.*, p. 541.
5. Margaret E. Hartford. *Groups in Social Work.* New York: Columbia University Press, 1971, p. 203.
6. Robert F. Bales. *Interaction Process Analysis.* Reading, Mass.: Addison-Wesley, 1950.
7. R. J. Patti, *op. cit.*, p. 543.
8. *Ibid.*, p. 544.
9. Catherine Papell and Beulah Rothman. Relating the Mainstream Model of Social Work with Groups to Group Psychotherapy and the Structured Group Approach. *Social Work with Groups, 3* (Summer 1980), pp. 5-23.

BOOK REVIEWS

THE CHALLENGE OF PARTNERSHIP: WORKING WITH PARENTS OF CHILDREN IN FOSTER CARE. Edited by Anthony Maluccio and Paula A. Sinanoglu. *New York: Child Welfare League of America, 1981, 225 pages, paperback.*

The Challenge of Partnership is a book about social work practice in the complicated arena of foster care. Though the specific focus is on work with biological parents of children in care, in a general sense this well-organized collection of papers manages to crystallize evolving practice theory and new methods of service delivery currently changing the whole context of child welfare. The essential premise of the book is articulated by David Fanshel in his Foreword:

> Biological parents are at the heart of the problem of "drift" and "impermanency" so repeatedly identified in recent years as the dominant feature of a nationwide system encompassing 500,000 children in care. Simply put, parents are rarely offered services designed to build up on their strengths to enable them to restore their homes as viable abodes for their children. We have a long history in the United States of crassly neglecting these parents and treating most of them as if they are not potentially valuable resources for their offspring. Once the children enter care, the parents are likely to be treated as discardable. (p. ix)

Based on this point of view, Maluccio and Sinanoglu circulated in 1979 a nationwide "Call for Papers on Biological Parents and Foster Care." The present volume consists of 11 papers selected from a total of 50 received, as well as one paper each contributed by the editors. The common theme linking all 13 papers is meant to be "partnership," that is the

> shared premise that we should work with biological parents as

> partners, rather than noncontributors or adversaries, if we are to achieve the basic child welfare goal of a secure, stable and loving home for each child. (Introduction, p. xv)

Of course, it is one thing to state a unifying theme and quite another to select, edit, and organize 11 separate pieces so that the theme is consistently developed from start to finish. Yet it is precisely in this regard that *The Challenge of Partnership* is so successful. Maluccio and Sinanoglu have put together a real rarity—a book of readings wherein the various separate contributions work together so that the whole really does become more than the sum of the parts. There are some of the usual problems with collections—a few of the contributions appear to be warmed over versions of material published in more complete detail elsewhere, and there is some unevenness of format and writing style from article to article—yet these are overshadowed by the impressive range of the articles selected, by clear editing, and by the lucid organization of the volume as a whole.

The book is divided into four sections. Part I is Overview, consisting of a selective review of the literature on biological parents of children in the foster care system by Paula A. Sinanoglu and a conceptual essay by Anthony Maluccio. The Sinanoglu piece is a distillation of a much more extensive review previously published by the editors. (See Anthony Maluccio and Paula A. Sinanoglu, "Social Work with Parents of Children in Foster Care," *Child Welfare,* May 1981.) Both readings are especially timely given present developments in child welfare.

Sinanoglu's analysis in the present volume—summarizing attitudes toward parents as reflected in the literature, and identifying major issues and programmatic trends—sets the stage for the range of different topics presented in the rest of the book.

Much more directly, Maluccio's essay, "An Ecological Perspective on Practice with Parents of Children in Foster Care," also serves to define the whole book. The author's summary of concepts generated by the ecological perspective and the life model of social work practice is brief but very clear. The clarity of presentation here is no small achievement in itself. Based on these ecological concepts Maluccio defines "the challenge of partnership" with parents of children in care in terms of the need for a generally restructured orientation to child welfare practice. While many of the ideas he presents are not new, the sharply drawn implications for practice are direct, challenging, and unmistakable. The remaining 11 articles in the book are clearly organized to expand and/or exemplify practice implications outlined in this introductory essay.

Part II of *The Challenge of Partnership* is entitled "Focus on Parents," with four articles connected by the argument that the whole family—especially the biological parents—must replace the individual child as the focus of effective child welfare practice. Shirley Jenkin's paper "The Tie that Bonds" is based on her provocative work on "filial deprivation," including conclusions from the longitudinal child welfare research conducted at the Columbia University School of Social Work and previously reported in more detail elsewhere.

The Janet Lahti and Jacquelyn Dvorak article, "Coming Home from Foster Care," focuses on the foster child's return home. Based on findings from the Oregon Project on Permanency Planning, Lahti and Dvorak suggest that the biological parents must be the focus of casework aimed at successful return home. The article describes a three-phase casework process with helpers and parents working together in each phase.

James K. Whittaker's "Family Involvement in Residential Treatment: A Support System for Parents" and Nadia Erlich Finkelstein's "Family-Centered Group Care—The Children's Institution, from a Living Center to a Center for Change" are both articles extending the implications of "partnership" to practice in children's institutions. The mere presence of two responses from the field of residential group care is indicative of how powerfully the ecological approach is beginning to shape practice in child welfare. Whittaker elegantly outlines both the historical problems and the real possibilities of parent involvement, redefining residential center as a family support system, rather than as a substitute form of care that treats the child in isolation from his family and home community. In more practical detail, Finkelstein defines and articulates "family-centered group care" as it is being developed at the Parsons Child and Family Center, Albany, New York. Her orientation to the realities of on-line practice is especially useful.

Part III is composed of articles describing four different practice approaches with biological parents of children in foster care. The focus of all four is on the parents, though the treatment orientations of the practitioners differ significantly. Eileen D. Gambrill and Theodore J. Stein's paper "Decision Making and Case Management: Achieving Continuity of Care for Children in Out-of-Home Placement" is the richest, most detailed piece in the collection.

Based on approaches developed in the famous Alameda Project, the authors describe an empirical approach to child welfare practice on behavioral intervention and early, mutual decision making by workers and parents. Ronald H. Rooney's "A Task-Centered Reunification Model for Foster" accepts the same necessity for empirical practice and early decision making, but utilizes task-centered approaches. In "Permanency Planning in Foster Care with the Ambivalent Parent," Arlene D. Jackson and Michael J. Dunne utilize psychodynamic concepts in formulating a time-limited counseling approach with biological parents. Finally, Rosemarie Carbino's "Developing a Parent Organization: New Roles for Parents of Children in Substitute Care" is a fascinating case study of social work practice as "network building," and advocacy. With its emphasis on supportive group and community work, the Carbino paper should be of special interest to readers of *Social Work with Groups.*

Part IV, "Foster Parent Roles," contains the final three selections. All of these articles focus on foster parents in redefined relationships with biological parents. Patricia Ryan, Emily Jean McFadden, and Bruce L. Warren's "Foster Families: A Resource for Helping Parents" acknowledges that not all foster parents can work with biological parents, yet still advocates viewing foster parents as part of the professional team rather than as part of a client system. This extension of the role of foster parent as family helper is briefly amplified in Edwin Johnston and Peter Gabor's "Parent Counselors: A Foster Care Program with New Roles for Major Participants," and also in James R. Seaberg's paper "Foster Parents as Aides to Parents." Unfortunately, though the concept of redefining roles and role expectations is consistent with an orientation to "ecological" intervention, this last section is the weakest in terms of detail and specific practice guidelines.

In the aggregate, all 13 papers in *The Challenge of Partnership* constitute a very valuable contribution to the practice literature. Professor Maluccio and his colleagues at the University of Connecticut School of Social Work have reinforced their standing among the most lucid, most well-informed voices in the rising chorus of advocates for reform of child welfare service delivery in the United States.

Richard W. Small, PhD
Assistant Professor
School of Social Welfare
State University of New York at Albany

BOARD MEMBERS ARE CHILD ADVOCATES: A PLAN FOR ACTION. Alan S. Gratch. *New York: Child Welfare League of America, 1980, 41 pages, paper.*

Mr. Gratch, a lawyer currently teaching at Loyola University in Chicago, has written an articulate and informative monograph based in part on his experiences as a board member of several social welfare agencies in the Chicago area. He states his thesis succinctly: "Each person who accepts a position on the board of directors of a child welfare agency automatically and without formality assumes the role of child advocate" (page 1). He points out that frequently, board members, and child welfare agencies in particular, may be in a better position to see other dimensions of policies and services and often have the position, knowledge and power to engage in advocacy more effectively than do others in an agency.

After presenting a theoretical justification for the board's advocacy function the author goes beyond ideological stance and exhortation to point out some of the problems and limitations of advocacy and in doing so, hopes to avoid the pitfalls of the sincere but sometimes uninformed, less skilled and ineffective advocacy efforts of the 1960s. Yet our debt to those who led the way is clear.

The material covered provides less of the "how-to" and more of the content of advocacy—the roles and functions of advocates and possible benefits on both local and broader levels. The roles and contributions of some of the actors other than board members are noted; "channels for advocacy activities" include legislative change, systems change, community education, and funding among others. However, I would have liked to see perhaps a little more of the particular difficulties in being an advocate in one's own agency as a preface to broader advocacy programs.

This is a most timely monograph in view of current political, judicial, and fiscal developments in child welfare programs and should be read not only by board members but by agency staffs as well. It is an excellent contribution and one which might be very helpful in restoring and impelling advocacy programs—a traditional and time honored function of voluntary agencies, particularly child welfare agencies.

Sherman Barr, DSW
Associate Professor of Social Work
New York University School of Social Work

CHILD ABUSE: PREVENTION AND TREATMENT THROUGH SOCIAL GROUP WORK. Julianne L. Wayne and Nancy C. Avery. *Boston, Mass.: Charles River Books, 1980, 81 pages.*

Those of us who, in the past four or five years, have read Wayne and Avery's articles on group services in the prevention and treatment of child abuse, met with anticipation the news that the authors were publishing a book on this subject, as the articles had provided a host of ideas on effective group programs for potential or actual non-nurturing parents and well-documented insights into the differential use of groups with this population. It is a little disappointing, therefore, to find out that the book does not amount to much more than a collection of these previous works. Nonetheless, it will be of great interest and use to social workers who deal with abusive or neglectful parents and who may not have easy access to the articles.

After the inevitable first chapter, here mercifully brief, on the history of child abuse, and a succinct one on its causes, Wayne and Avery offer their views on "The Special Value of Social Group Work" to alleviate the problem. It is in this chapter that, presumably, the theoretical underpinnings of their practice are set forth. As it turns out, the authors do not do themselves justice here: by borrowing Yalom's schema of "curative factors" and relying nearly exclusively on these in lieu of a rationale for using groups, they neglect the embryonic "conceptual map" that was present in their already published work and to which Kolodny refers in his Foreword. In these articles, the authors had started to pull together strands from various theories: that of Garland, Jones and Kolodny on the stages of group development, that of Kubler-Ross and others on grief work or therapy, and that of Middleman on the purposeful and differential use of activities. Yet another strand which runs through their practice, and which provides the basis for a later chapter, is Reiner and Kaufman's theory on character disordered clients. All these strands are still waiting to be forged into a strong and coherent theoretical whole. The adoption of "Yalom's ten," though it provides interesting insights into the possibilities of group help for this particular population, distracts the authors from opening the new theoretical frontiers which their earlier work promised.

The next four chapters are made up of the articles referred to above. They are very good. First, one learns about the successful implementation of a group work program in a protective agency. The authors stress that different clients need different groups, and they discuss a number of alternatives: a "remedial" discussion group, a socialization group, and a task-oriented group. Then the "remedial" group is analyzed in terms of grief work with the depressed and the angry, who make up most of the non-nurturing population. This is an excellent piece of work, illustrating the best in social work practice—a deep sense of caring about people, a disciplined use of self, an application of the theories of human behavior, and a discriminating use of practice theory, in this case social work with groups. In the course of this group's experience, the authors introduced activities in the pretermination phase. This is detailed in another chapter and offers added proof of Wayne and Avery's professional creativity.

Because abusive parents are not only depressed and angry individuals, but also are socially isolated, they constitute a hard-to-reach population. It is therefore very useful to find in the book an account of an outreach program designed to prevent child maltreatment. Moreover, if it is true that government funds for child welfare are being diverted from foster care to prevention, this short description of a successful program should become required reading for mental health professionals working in protection.

Finally, the point that non-nurturing parents need a range of services is well-made, both in a chapter discussing two specific abusive families and in the conclusion.

Despite some limitations, this book provides a thoughtful and practice-tested guide to preventing child abuse and helping non-nurturing parents through the use of social group work. Social workers who want to intervene more effectively with their clients, whether these are abusive or neglectful of their children, or simply non-trusting, depressed and angry individuals, will learn much from reading it.

Margot Breton
Faculty of Social Work
University of Toronto

THE RESIDENTIAL COMMUNITY. Howard Jones. *London: Routledge and Kegan Paul, 1979, 145 pages.*

How can a reviewer take exception to any portion of a book on social work in which appear marvelously crisp comments like, "As the old saying goes, 'one volunteer is worth two pressed men' "? Is it really possible to maintain a detached and critical stance when an author, in the midst of a discussion of the role of volunteers on British residential staffs, conjures up visions of eighteenth-century press gangs, bringing back delightful memories of seafaring tales out of one's youth? When, after all, was the last time that an American reader, perusing a chapter on housing arrangements in children's homes, came across a lovely aphorism like "temper the wind to the shorn lamb," or encountered a professional text in which words like "tetchiness" were unself-consciously used by the writer, and to good effect?

As literature, *The Residential Community* is a treat. It seems fair to say that in the United States we are not accustomed to as urbane and graceful a style in books on social work, or indeed on any of the helping professions, as one finds in this volume. "Well-crafted" is the phrase which comes immediately to mind.

Urbanity, however, is not the chief attraction of *The Residential Community.* For this reviewer, at least, its most attractive feature is the artful manner in which its author, Howard Jones, impresses on the reader's attention the philosophical dilemmas which lie at the heart of social work in all custodial institutions and helps him to think them through. This is particularly true of the conflict between the professional's commitment to the institutionalized client and his commitment to societal norms and demands which the client may disavow. This is a slim volume, but the writer of many a larger work on the same subject has blinked at the prospect of discussing this conflict and ended by considering it only briefly and with little enthusiasm. Here the author's thoughts on the matter are given great play in several chapters. This is most helpful to those social work practitioners in residential settings, whether group workers, caseworkers or administrators, who think and feel beyond technique, to questions of purpose and ethics.

Jones, who is professor of social administration at University College, Cardiff, is concerned with institutions offering any one of three major categories of long-term care. These may be institutions which conceive of themselves as asylums, those which are designed to protect the public, and, finally, those which were created for the nurture of children who presumably would otherwise be deprived of appropriate nurturance. One is a first startled to observe three such different types of institutions—nursing homes, prisons, and children's residential treatment centers—being housed under one conceptual roof. At least in those sections of the book which deal with the impact of removal from home and society's expectations of the behavior of the inhabitants of any total institution, the device works. As a consequence of its use, the reader is helped to see, rather more clearly than he may have before, the similarities in the psychological demands made by all three of these institutions on both residents and staff.

Ten chapters comprise the book, each of them relatively brief, with discussion sharpened to point up what the author considers the most important issues under the topic at hand. The history and sociology of institutional treatment in Great Britain form the bedrock of the material which follows and is laid out in the first chapter. This is succeeded by analysis of the manner in which such institutions are organized and the philosophies behind various forms of organization, as well as their differential social and psychological impact. A third succinct chapter on "Justifications" is only eight pages long, but Jones packs into these pages enough thought-provoking material to keep the reader occupied for quite some time.

"Succinct" should not be confused with "superficial," especially in these early chapters of the book. In regard to "justifications," for instance, Jones asks, "What right do we have to disturb people's life-styles and relationships, especially in the drastic way that residential placement entails?" He then goes on to wrestle with this question vigorously, avoiding none of the value conflicts it poses for the social worker. Easy rationalizations are not for this author. He is no more completely satisfied with social work's conception of deviant behavior as "sickness" than he is with notions of deviance as moral turpitude. Our purpose in conceiving of deviance as psychological illness, after all, may largely stem from our need to justify "treating" this "disease" by means of the quasi-medical model we have adopted from the psychotherapies. Not a new point, surely. The reader's perspective, however, is enlarged, first, by the manner in which Jones examines this issue from every side, and, second, by the sensible way in which he resolves the matter for himself. He emphasizes the notion of a contract which acknowledges that social workers and clients may sometimes have different aims in mind regarding how it would be best for the client to act, but assumes that they can reach a *modus vivendi*. In this connection, clients' perception of their needs are taken seriously. At the same time, although workers' belief that, because of their training, they can distinguish between the felt "wants" of clients and their "needs," i.e., what they should have for their own good, is patronizing and authoritarian, it must be said that this proposition may nevertheless be true. The psychodynamic approach to understanding verbal as well as other behavior, Jones emphasizes—and he makes excellent use of such understanding himself—has considerable validity. Clearly, there are cases, he reminds us, where accepting clients' first statements may be to their disadvantage.

Throughout this seminal chapter on justifications, Jones continues to wrestle with these notions in this manner. "So even if one rejects the view that the dominant culture is always right, with its accompanying 'sickness assumption,' " he concludes, "it does not follow, either, that the client is always right. How to reconcile such a discovery with the idea of the social work contract is not easy. There is no way in which one can justify the social worker's dictating to clients, but at least he has to be given time to convince them that they have got it wrong." Disturbing someone's life-style, as social workers do, whether the person in question is prisoner, nursing home resident or child in residential placement, may represent the enforcement or inducement of conformity. But, says Jones, the enforcement of conformity is justified if it is undertaken by "a legitimately constituted authority acting against a serious threat to the common interest." Jones suggests the residential social worker in his groups or individual interviews avoid manipulating people into conformity and face honestly the element of compulsion involved. His view is that we will then be clear about how great a threat to the general interest needs to be to justify the use by the social worker of such pressure to conform.

Of the remaining chapters, those dealing with such matters as "Order," "Selection," "Relationships" and "Change" amplify and give body to this point of view. This is where *The Residential Community* is at its strongest, articulating a philosophy and indicating the directions in which an administrator and staff should move if this philosophy is to be "lived out" in actual practice.

Less satisfying are the chapters on "Programme" and "Staffing." Here, brevity of discussion, and the treatment of all three types of institutions as versions of a single residential form falter as literary and conceptual devices. One does better, for example, to read Fritz Redl, whom Jones cites, and the work of Albert Trieschman and James Whittaker for insights into the use of program activities and staff tensions in residential work with children. Similarly, related issues in prison work are subjected to a more detailed analysis in the writings of someone like Seymour Hallet. (It should be added, by the way, that Jones' British prisons come through as rather tame places by American standards.) In this sense *The Residential Community* is best thought of as an *introduction* to social work in the residential institution. As such, however, it is an excellent representative of the genre. This reviewer recommends it earnestly to his fellow group workers.

Ralph Kolodny, MA, MSW
Professor
Boston University School of Social Work

AUDIO-VISUAL REVIEW

There was an announcement in the last issue of *Social Work with Groups* of the inauguration of an audio-visual review section to be edited by Lawrence Shulman.

What could be more appropriate in launching this section than a review of one of Larry's videotapes?

Persons interested in having tapes reviewed may contact: Lawrence Shulman, Professor, School of Social Work, University of British Columbia, Vancouver, B.C. V6T 1W5.

LEADING A FIRST SESSION. Lawrence Shulman. *McGill University, Montreal. $225.00 (rental—Syracuse University, NY, $50.00) 3/4" cassettes, in color.*

In this videotape Lawrence Shulman has highlighted themes central to group life—the authority of the worker and the potential for establishing interdependence in the group—as these themes are manifest in first sessions. Juxtaposing sequences from Shulman's own practice with a couple's group and his didactic sessions with social work students, Shulman models a caring, skilled and self-reflecting practitioner as well as a thoughtful, theoretically grounded and authentic teacher. This ninety minute two-reel tape has relevance for the beginning practitioner as well as the seasoned and theoretically sophisticated worker.

Both in his practice and in his teaching Shulman's awareness of the group worker's feelings and perceptions as guides to intervention is vividly illustrated. As a result, this tape presents visual support for utilizing self-awareness to understand the nuances of specific situations and to enhance practice theory in general.

The group, conducted in a psychiatric setting, is composed of five couples with various psychiatric histories. However, Shulman's introduction of members to the viewers within their social context rather than in terms of their clinical maladies, develops the broader social work perspective that these are not simply carriers of chronic illness but people seeking help with their lives. Shulman thus establishes the purpose of the mutual aid system and guides its development as a group that can support change.

The disparity in group members' ages points up a simple truth regarding group composition, mainly that common ground, in this case, marital problems, constitutes the most significant compositional variable. The film demonstrates Shulman's vision of the group as "a living passages" generating grist for the mill, rather than an intergenerational system encumbered by communication problems.

Throughout the film Shulman highlights salient issues and teaches important practice principles. For example, he sanctions as valid the worker's rehearsal of opening statements to the group. In beginning the group, he makes a straightforward statement about group purpose which focuses members on what is—that these couples have experienced some problems in the past—and asks them to share what they would like to change. His simple statement engages members' motivation for beginning.

Another important practice principle emerges from examining the participation of Ben, a pivotal group member, who prototypically talks for his wife. Shulman stops the group tape and engages in a didactic exchange with students involving a professional discussion of whether or not to interrupt a member. The principle of "creating safety in the group" is established as the couple's defenses are accepted not challenged.

Ben's behavior in the first session is also prototypic to group members. He challenges the power of the authority figure indirectly by talking at length about how ineptly psychiatrists have interacted with him in the past. He poses a threat that could provoke a worker's anger at his challenge to the professional's competence. Shulman accepts Ben; doesn't attack him or engage in a power struggle with him. Nor does he overly identify with Ben's dominated wife. To the students he teaches that "people with anger are not your enemies; they want to work." Shulman establishes the inherent right to question the role of the worker within the relationship itself. He creates a broad inclusion norm that enables Ben to be a creative contributing member not a deviant. He models the principle of "scanning the group,"—noting how members are reacting to other's participation—and recognizes that "Ben is speaking for others in the group in reflecting some of their feelings about prior helpers."

Throughout the film Shulman makes a point about mutuality and reciprocity in all helping processes. He points practitioners and students in the direction toward tuning in and sustaining empathy. He tells the students "I try to feel what it's like to be them."

Many problems are presented as members, responding to Ben's leadership, begin to test the waters and experience the group's potential, some now talking about their own negative experiences with other helpers. Because Ben is able to get past his concern with authority he is able to lead. Since Shulman is able to handle his own authority he fosters an attitude that allows others to lead. Ben takes over the helping role, going around the group and drawing members out. The worker does not compete with Ben; rather at times he augments Ben's emerging leadership and enables the process. In teaching, Shulman further clarifies saying "When they began to feel it was their group, I began to relax."

In reflecting about his own practice in this film, Shulman shares his dissatisfaction with how he handled Ben's initial concern about helpers, admitting that he got "uptight" with the presenting challenge. He articulates another important set of principles. There is no "right" or "wrong" in the interactive process that unfolds. Effectiveness in communication is not absolute but defined in the unfolding situation. Yet another reflective piece in the process involves the value of silence as a tool for workers, which Shulman aptly demonstrates.

And so from start to finish we encounter in this tape exemplary practice and conceptually clear teaching developed in an authentic and unpretentious manner. Viewers are left with faith in their capacities to develop "non-mystical" skills. Moreover, from these principles, in conclusion they may have gained awareness of perhaps the most distinguished principles of social group work as represented by Shulman's impactful words:

"Who owns the group? *They* do."

"Who runs the group? *They* do."

Urania Glassman, MA, MSW
Assistant Director
Field Work
New York University School of Social Work

CALL FOR PAPERS

Special Edition of *Social Work with Groups:* "Time-Limited Groups."

Under the Dual Guest Editorship of A.S. Alissi and Max Casper.

You are invited to submit manuscripts dealing with different aspects of social group work practice, theory and research on time-limited group experiences:

* The use of short-term frames in practice
* The single session group experience
* On-going group structures with changing memberships
* Differential use of skills, techniques and methods in long-term, short-term and single session groups

Manuscript is due by September 1, 1983.

Manuscripts may be submitted to the Guest Editors or to the Editors of *Social Work with Groups.* Please refer to Instructions for Authors.

Albert S. Alissi, University of Connecticut, School of Social Work, Greater Hartford Campus, West Hartford, Conn. 06117.

Max Casper, Syracuse University, School of Social Work, Brockway Hall, Syracuse, New York 13210.